Walking the Recovery Road: The Steps Taken

by Melody Rose Paul

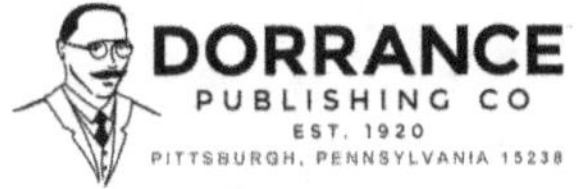

DORRANCE
PUBLISHING CO
EST. 1920
PITTSBURGH, PENNSYLVANIA 15238

Dorrance Publishing Co
585 Alpha Drive
Suite 103
Pittsburgh, PA 15238
Visit our website at *www.dorrancebookstore.com*

ISBN: 979-8-8868-3203-7
eISBN: 979-8-8868-3776-6

After coming back to Bangor, I realized how lucky I was to be alive and free from those walls of the Maine state prison. Once I stepped foot on United States' soil again, I realized just how lucky I was to be a Native American and to be able to exercise my rights as a Native to freely cross the United States/ Canadian border. I am very proud of my native blood, and I want to be able to change my situations and make my people proud.

When I arrived back in Bangor Maine, I was excited to get back to my apartment and just settle into a routine again. I went to the grocery store to get myself a few things that I would be needing for my first day at work… supplies and some ice cream. Yes, for some strange reason, I don't understand where it came from, but this unbelievable sweet tooth that I have today. I think it's since I've given up mostly everything that has to do with my pleasure senses. I like to think of sweets as my anxiety coping skill, my only small treat of every other day.

Starting my new routine consisted of early daily prayer, meditation, and exercise for the mind and soul. Also getting back into my Native culture and beliefs with smudge with sage. My spirituality has been the most affected /damaged by my substance use over the years.

I noticed things more as my mind cleared itself of substance daily, I grew stronger and clearer headed as the days went by. I knew that I needed to focus on my responsibilities as a parent. That was my official drive to not look back at any negative situations that I had caused myself and others.

On the first day of my new job at the "coffee shop," I decided to walk instead of taking a taxicab or city bus, just to clear my mind and ease my high anxiety. I've always had a bit of anxiety when starting a new place of employment. It didn't matter where it was. I just knew that I had a long day ahead of me and I needed to focus on doing well and not walking off the job on the first day. Trust and believe me when I say that I've walked off a job thirty minutes into it.

My first day as a barista, I didn't know how to run most of the machines that my new boss, Joe, wanted me to figure out. I got very overwhelmed, but I didn't allow it to ruin my day. I waited until the right moment to approach my new coworkers. I knew that it could be difficult, so I was careful. I was introduced to Loretta. I hit it off with her instantly. It was like I had already known her for years. We instantly connected. She also gave me the pointers that I needed to make the drinks properly. Loretta made me feel comfortable and welcome there. Loretta has this energy about her that makes people comfortable, almost like motherly, which I though was nice. I didn't spill any drinks or have no complaints that day.

My first day back to work wasn't as bad as my addict mind thought. I did seriously think that I would end up spilling a drink accidently on a customer or some of my coworkers. I knew mixing drinks all day wasn't too bad. I had taken a coffee job before in my early twenties. Back then I was so irresponsible and carefree that I worked long enough to save a bit of money then leave. Insanity at its best.

My workdays became routine after a few weeks went by and "the crew" made me feel welcome and I felt that they had a bit of respect for me. Loretta became my favorite coworker at the shop. She was always someone that I knew I could talk to and be honest with. She would call me Miss MEL and I didn't mind it. It reminded me of the days when I was seventeen working in the blueberry fields back in Washington County. Loretta was from the county and that is why I felt an instant connection with her. She had recently lost her husband. She told me how much she loved him, and my heart just melted over that. I listened to her talk about how difficult of a life change that was for her and honestly, I could not imagine that kind of pain and loss.

Those first few weeks at the coffee shop. I was learning how to not only make regular coffee but expresso coffees, lattes, and fruit mixes, which was a science all on its own. One of the sassy ladies that I worked with was Jure. Jure, being so street smart was like some of the women I was in prison with. She would, like, sense when I was annoyed. It was from her street-smart ways that she could always tell when I became frustrated. She would stop me and say "Melody, just breath, girl." I would listen to her, and she would help me finish my iced macchiatos. Jure became one of the ladies that helped me regularly when I needed a "time out" minute. She was always there to watch over me when I was making large orders, sometimes she would smile and wait for me until I needed her help. She had a way about her that always stood out to everyone, and the customers loved her. Sometimes at the end of each shift she would be so ready to leave that she would get silly and sing to the customers. That always made me laugh. Jure, I do thank you. I love you girl.

Another one of my favorites at the coffee shop was Tabatha. She had this boldness about her that I admire about people on the daily. Tabby, as everyone liked to call her, was also an ex-Windham (mcc) gal as well. When things got hectic with customers or workers. She wanted to make me laugh. She would mention a mcc slang that only her and I would understand. We bonded very quickly over our past struggles. I noticed a tatt on her neck that said, "One day at a time." We started talking to each other about our old addictive sick ways and how lucky we were to be one of the few who were able to find recovery. I enjoyed our mini meetings at work, and I also want to thank Tabatha for the support.

I also instantly connected to Shawn G; he trained me properly and schooled me up on the ways of the store and the special drinks. Tricks and trades, as you will. He had been working there for five years and knew a lot about everything and he always was there when I would get a bunch of early morning sometimes grumpy and not so friendly customers.

Customer service can be tricky at times, especially in early recovery; wow, what a challenge I placed myself in. I had no clue as to how fast-paced it would be at times. One of the first few customers that I made coffees for was this regular named Barbara, she had this energy about her that fueled the fires around her. She knew that I had recently just got hired and was polite to me and encouraged me to not let the other workers or customers bother me. Her advice honestly helped me get through some of the not-so-easy days at the coffee shop.

After a few weeks I started to get to know the regulars and I enjoyed making drinks and I did not even mind the fast pace of the store. This store was busy. The line in the morning would be wrapped right around drive-through, also an extensive line out the front door.

Being around people that wanted to work and be addicted to coffee instead of any other substance made it extremely easy to adapt to as well. I started to allow myself to get to know my coworkers and customers and it helped me to feel more stress free. I was always alone in those first few months at my tiny apartment only made for one person and a pet, lol. It was home and a job and that's all that I cared about at the time. I was stable with a routine and healthy working environment, which is all that I cared for at the time.

My first three months of sobriety were hard. I managed to not "slip up" as some people like to call it. I just plain and simple avoided people that I knew would easily trigger me. I did not give a lot of my time to allow people in anyway. The places that I knew where I could easily get temptations would be the first avoided areas—bars, small outdoor gatherings, social events, etc.

I shut it down when I would "bump into old party (using friends). I became the shutdown queen in my mind. I would be either walking home from work or going to a meeting, then suddenly, I would hear "Hey, Melody how you been?" I look to see who it was and sure enough someone that I partied with. I got in my awkward/antisocial mode, then would politely answer "Oh hey, I am doing good, I'm clean and sober again and I am staying that way." They usually would give me a strange look and just say "That's good…good for you." Although there was some that would like to encourage me and be like, "Melody, you look good when you're being good and staying to yourself." I was flattered at times, sometimes I had a slight temptation to lose my composure…lose my SH**.

The funny thing is, that I enjoyed being clean from substance and without the need of a drink to feel good in my skin. Walking to work in the early mornings sure did help me get into a "can't kill my mood" kind of mode. The natural high that I would get from daily exercise was one of the things that I did regularly to get me in the right frame of mind. I would, like, sort out my addiction thoughts, and I would pray instead. I needed the guidance as well from a higher power, so I started to walk/pray/meditative state of calm and easy to myself kind of mood. My spirituality helped me to be able to have an unclouded vision of what I needed to accomplish every day. Goals that I set for myself were daily challenges for me to overcome. One of the goals that I had set up for myself was to publish my 90,000 words that I had on a flash drive that was not completed yet.

The memoir that I had written while I was incarcerated, imprisoned for one of my self-seeking and sick behaviors. I thought about getting it published, but I was not sure the process. I knew that I had invested many hours sitting down to type up a life story that was full of crazy adventures with some brutally honest situations. I was healing from my crazy life and in those first three months I knew that I could not fill my plate too much because it would overflow, so I put the book on hold to focus on my recovery.

Once again, I started the process of court proceedings for custody/reunification with my son, Anthony. It was one of the major causes of my relapse. I wanted to tackle it head-on with nothing in my way, especially my sickness. I knew that in the years before, I had an obligation to be there for this young man…I wanted to have him around me. I missed a whole two years with him.

Due to the protection from harassment order on me, I knew that I needed to have that amended at first challenge. I knew that from what I had been through before with my ex would make things difficult for me once again. Unfortunately, I knew that deep down I was going to have a challenge getting custody of my son again. I started attending more meetings and I reached out to people that I knew were living a clean and healthy lifestyle.

I was able to reach out to one of the ladies at the domestic violence center. I knew the place well because I was present at a few of their support groups for a least a year straight. I learned a lot about how to cope not only with what I was going through at the time, but how I could be helpful to others as well.

I wanted and needed the services that are provided at this center, I was able to get a volunteer advocate to help me file the proper court papers for visits and reunification with Anthony, what my legal rights and responsibilities were as a parent. I knew that my son needed his mother for support, and I made it one of my main goals and placed it on my priority list.

I know firsthand the heartache that comes with a missing parent. Although my stepfather, Keith, was able to fill that void most of my life, I still had this empty feeling inside. Slightly neglected, during my childhood made me aware of things that I should have never had to face as a youth. I did not want my son to experience that same kind of neglectfulness and mental turmoil that I had went through. I wanted to be a healthy version of myself, the way I was meant to be before substance ruined my life. I had a profound respect for this domestic violence center in Bangor. They had helped me several times before and they knew me. I had done some classes there before and I went to the weekly support group for a year straight.

I was able to get a lady to help me file the proper papers for custody/visits and I filed the paperwork as soon as I had a free afternoon. The paperwork was filed and then the waiting process started. It only took a short couple of weeks to get in to speak with the judge. I had prepared myself well this time. I had all my certificates from the prison from the many classes I had taken. Honestly, prison does not have to be a waste of time. The state's able to provide enough recourse to remain busy and productive. So, if you know someone in jail or prison that say there's nothing to do…well, that is a straight lie. I had taken about six self-help groups, which usually last about a six- to eight-week span, depending on the class really.

So, I had a file folder with me. When it was time to enter the courtroom to ask for visits. I had a stable job, an apartment, a community of supportive people that I was learning to trust as well. I had a slight relapse with drinking that lasted for about two weeks and nothing like before. I was only able to bounce back because I knew that I did not want to live foolishly anymore.

When it came time for us to speak to the judge to amend order, I was a bit scared but confident because I knew that I was not the same person as before the order was granted. I was changing for the better and I was hopeful for the future. A positive mindset and a program that I started to utilize instead of running away from. I was in a different frame of mind now. I had no interest in fighting with anyone except for what I knew deep down was the right thing to do, that was fighting for my rights to be the mother that I knew I could be.

The judge asked who wanted to start and I was all for it, so that I knew what strategy to use as a defense. My ex started to talk negatively about me, he also included how my "family" was also unhealthy and unkind, which is not true at all. He mentioned things from my past from years prior and thought in his sick mind that my son would be better off without a mother that could not change. This went on for about twenty minutes. He insulted me and my whole family. His deep resentment towards me was still so fresh and obviously very resentful.

My force was to be as kind and honest as I could be. I wanted to let the judge know firsthand that I was in recovery and that I was attending daily meetings. I said in my testimony that I had an apartment and that I had started working at the coffee shop a few months prior and that I was able to pay my rent and continue with my recovery process with the help of a twelve-step program and support from the local community center (Bangor Area Recovery Network). I had recently just offered my time to the barn to clean the building and take phone calls, so I did mention that as well. This, my friends, is called "service work."

The judge asked if we might "have anything else to add before I decide?" I had nothing to add because I had already passed in all the proof of the months of classes and changes that I had accepted. I was ready to be a parent; I was ready for my son. Then my ex said he wanted to add a few more things…he continued with his insults and negativity towards me, and I just had nothing to say because I did not care about what he thought of me anymore. I knew that I was trying my best and I also knew that my son needed a mother.

The judge looked at both of us and he took a deep breath then said, "I honestly cannot even believe that this order was granted in the first place." I was so surprised and happy in my heart. The months I tried so hard to get visits at the prison with my son and just to be able to have him in my life once again was a good moment for me. The judge said I will not amend order. I am going to dismiss it because it's not right to keep an order on someone that's clearly not a danger to her son. He also congratulated my progress and wished me good luck on my journey, and he said nothing to my ex. I do consider this one of my promises of my early months of recovery. It was a moment that I first realized that I could start to really take some accountability for my past negative and self-sabotaging behavior…to move forward from my past.

My journey was only starting, and I knew that this was one for the books. Later that night I waited for Charlie to call me from the prison, and I was so excited to tell him that the order was finally dropped…after two long years. I could almost predict what time Charlie would call, the phone would ring at usually seven or seven thirty. A lady with a sweet tone would be on the other end (Prison Operator recording) saying "you have a free call from Charles M." I also knew how long each call would be, approximately fifteen minutes. Charlie became one of my daily supports those early months of sobriety. He always said how proud of me he was that I came back to my senses after my short relapse.

I was excited to talk to him and tell him that this time I was profoundly serious about changing my life around and that I was ready to be honest and live honestly. I also knew that there were challenges ahead of me that I would not be able to overcome if I was actively using any substance. Charlie was so excited when I told him the good news that I could start the visits in a matter of a few weeks. I was also so excited to share this moment/highlight together. After falling hard on my face and serving time for my insane behavior, I knew this was a turning point.

I was on a natural high from excitement for a few days after this. My regular routine of work, meetings and not socially isolating from my newfound friends in recovery. I knew that I needed a sponsor, someone that would be able to help guide me with the "steps." I already had someone in mind, someone that I knew from when I was in rehab back in 2012. The sad part about this is I wanted her to be my sponsor back in 2012, but I was mentally not ready to take responsibility for myself. Yes, that does happen, and it happened to me. I faked it and I fell hard on my face.

This time I felt ready. I was in getting clearer in my body mind and soul. I was getting comfortable talking about my daily life and about what I needed to continue for success. I was anxious but ready to ask her to help me. I see her at the community center, and I knew that was the time.

I said to her with a big smile, "HI, Ana, how are you? Do you remember me?"

She replied, "Of course I do, but enlighten me please." I opened to her and told her that I remembered her from the years before in rehab, but I did not have mental focus back then. She said to me, "I would be honored to help." She set up some weekly rules with me. I was to follow these rules for success. Number one was never saying something and not following through; number two was always being on time for our weekly hour check-in meeting. Number three is home group and service. I was game, I needed to be accountable for myself and she would be a "guider" for me in my newfound freedom and I was ready. Ana has this powerful positive energy that I just love and admire about her. Honestly even today as I draft this story, I know I must check in with her today.

Then after weeks of working at the coffee shop and doing my self-care for my recovery process, I received a certified letter in the mail. I knew it was coming, so I was not nervous about it but excited. I knew it was a step closer to changing my parental rights. It was to modify child custody order and child support order. I had a date to appear in court and I was more than ready. I had that disease of addiction in my head as well saying, *"you need to comfort and cope so come back to me."* I did not want to drink or use substance. I didn't want to "numb out." I wanted to feel even the pain of any rejection, any happiness, any anxiety as well. So, I called a sober friend and called Ana, then went to the meeting that night.

I was afraid to face the realization that I could only have my son on the weekends or every other weekend. I had full parental rights with him for thirteen years. I knew my son. I wanted to be there daily for him, the reality of my situation was "baby steps" to progress.

I had to accept that there was a chance that I would only be allowed weekly visits and that I did not have the control that I once had as a parent. I was in a different state of mind this time, I was in recovery. I prepared myself in the weeks before my court date because I knew it could be good or bad for me. I did everything that I knew would help me and not hurt me. Before when a court date would not work in my favor. I would go on a massive self-sabotage "bender." I knew to keep myself in check.

When the court date finally arrived, I walked down to the courthouse with nervous energy but also, I was ready, actually more than ready to have my son back in my life. I was lonely. I usually was alone because I have no family in Maine. I only have my son and it hurt when I could not see him. I believe that some people are so sick and angry that they would go to the extreme to cause hurt and discontent. I walked into the courtroom, and I noticed that nobody was there except for us and a few of the court workers. The process took about thirty minutes to agree for weekly visits to start immediately. I was so excited about it. I was able to have every Saturday with the option to sleep over when I was ready. Honestly, I was not close to ready for overnights yet, I was barely ready for weekly.

I also was ordered to pay child support, which luckily enough for me was by income limitations, so I did not have to pay too much so that I could keep up with my other bills. Luckily, I was given a time to organize my work schedule to fit in my days with my son, it worked out perfectly. At first it was nice to have him be dropped off at the coffee shop. I would usually get him a small latte with a Boston cream or strawberry with sprinkles. I would work the extra hour, then we usually would check out stores in the area or hit the gym together for a few. I have to say that it was nice to be able to build a healthy relationship with my son again. Becoming the mother that he deserves was becoming our reality and that was a small miracle.

After a few weeks, I started the process of getting to know my son. I could not understand why he was so closed to me emotionally. Everything takes time I understand this now because I was able to slow down enough to see the transformation that I had started as well.

So far, I do understand that trusting someone into your space and soul is a lot. It took me many months as well to let anyone into my personal space. I think the time that it takes just to even get to know any person causes anxiety. Today I allow people in my world. My recovery mentally has been extremely helpful with me opening to anyone…also everyone like with my first book *Savaged to Wellness*.

Anyways after a few months, I felt happy in my soul again. Honestly, even just a weekly date (Saturdays) with my son made me feel the special mother glow that we all get. Honestly, I should say parent glow that we all get, because there are also some very awesome fathers that must go through hurdles as well.

I had also started to regularly attend the weekly Friday Wellbriety that was being held at "the Wab" as the local Natives like to call it, as do I as well. I started to get more involved in community service as well. I had a nice routine…a weekly routine. Very crucial, I might add to any recovery program. It is needed to survive our boredom as addictive people.

Meeting regularly with my sponsor, Ana, she encourages me to get into community service. I did not want to at first and I thought about being dishonest about it but knew that was a black road. Lies to cover lies and so on and so forth. The insanity could start again, and I wasn't about to get sucked into that. So, I called the local area recovery center to see if I could start my service work as soon as possible. I was desperate to continue this great path I had started to slowly rebuild. I was extremely nervous when they finally excepted me to become a weekly volunteer. On the day of my interview to get the service position, yes, I was nervous; I did not know what to say. I just remembered what Ana told me… "Just be yourself and you will be fine." That was all that I knew I needed. I would start my weekly service that following week. My supervisor at the coffee shop was very understanding and supported my recovery process, which at the time was immensely helpful for me. Honestly, having supportive positive people around you when you're just starting over is gold.

After a few weeks of showing up for my Wednesday-afternoon position at the recovery center, I felt a sense of warmth from my new friends that I was making them. I would look forward to seeing the regulars playing their card games of poker or cribbage after meetings. I would be friendly as if I were still working, serving coffee for the community. I would welcome people as they entered the building. I also was required to do some physical chores as well. Cleaning, sweeping the floors, cleaning bathrooms as well as taking out the trash. I did not mind it one bit…it made me feel good inside.

I was still alone at the Ohio Street apartment and, honestly, I was very lonely at times. I kept a lot to myself because I was scared to allow anyone to enter my space. My safe area, which I will call it, my sobriety circle, the imaginary bubble that I had created to keep myself safe from the dangers of addiction. The service work provided me a safe clean environment. A place that I could slowly let down my guard. I was happy to be at the recovery center and work.

Anything that would help me stay occupied during the "Lonely Months" of my recovery process. Lonely because I slept alone, walked every place alone, ate alone, etc. I was okay inside, though; I was healing. Occasionally, I would do different things like get on a bus and travel to down east Maine to visit just for the day. But really, I knew that could be a trigger to "party mode," so I stayed on my recovery path. I stayed local in my area, close to home and gravitated to mostly recovery people. It was like I was starting a new family or new relationship with a mate; except I was not. I was just starting the process of healing my soul…my damaged soul. I was good and things were starting to slowly take place in my life.

I was starting to get to know people, only because I became vulnerable. I opened my soul in my weekly recovery meeting, and I allowed the process of healing to take place. I stayed accountable to everything I did, and I was honest in all my affairs. I knew that I could not afford to relapse into that cold depression of drunkenness or numbing feelings like I use to. I knew I could lose everything that I was actively working towards…goals. I used to think that I did not deserve to have a stable home, decent job, education, sober/ clean meaningful relationships. It was a great feeling to know that if I got in a situation that I could just pick up my phone and call someone that was in recovery, and they would just listen to me vent. Also, to encourage and remind me of why we addicts should never bow down to our lowest point and break. There was a constant reminder of what I could easily become again while living at the Ohio Street apartment. There were regular drinking parties downstairs on the first floor. I would hear them screaming and singing sometimes all night during the weekends. I would also smell several types of smells in the halls when entering my place. It would be difficult for me to relax sometimes, but I knew the times when they would shut music off, usually around ten, then I could sleep.

There were also people that worked in the building, so I would be able to rest before those early morning shifts at the coffee shop. I started to focus on my physical health as well as my mental health. I joined a local gym; I created a workout schedule. I wanted to look and feel well. I hit the gym usually daily, usually before or after the nightly recovery meeting…my medicine.

I started to get to know the people in the building. They would see that I was busy usually and I would politely say hello and nod my head. I would lock both locks in my apartment at night and I always tried to be quiet so I would be left alone as well. I wanted to be left alone and they did not bother. Everyone in the building knew that I was clean and sober…I mean I did not even smoke.

I was lonely during the evenings, but that was also the time that I knew Charlie would call me. Usually, the same time every night. I almost knew when the phone would ring, I had a certain ring tone on my cell phone that would go off when it was Charlie. It would play a harmonica ring. That is when I knew my best friend was on the other line. He was in that dark cold place still serving his time, and I was getting a head start on life. I knew that I wanted to build a healthier life. I wanted a healthy life with Charlie. I also could understand that people do make mistakes and I was not about to abandon Charlie. He was there for me when I went through the pain of not having my son daily. But also, Charlie was also the reason I was tempted to first try a powerful drug called heroin. So, it was difficult for me to focus on trusting my heart with him. I honestly did not even know if I wanted to be in a serious relationship again. I, after all, was in this beautiful healing process…a "healing my inner core" process.

Recovery is tricky at times because you really do have to be careful of whom you decide to have in your inner circle—a "boundary balance," let us just call it. A space that you have built and worked so hard towards that you cannot allow anyone to destroy your brick walls. As always, I give people a chance and Charlie is just one of those souls that I happen to love. A connection since I first met him back when he picked me up in the old dirty rusty work truck.

Well, I would spend hours on the phone with him. I knew when that voice on the other end would say "you have a call from an inmate at department of corrections," I would ninety percent of the time be able to answer his call. We talked about our day count usually and what we missed about being together again. I told him that I would wait for him and that I would get a larger apartment and get prepared for when he was released from prison. I told him that I would have everything that he needed. It was months away, this meant that I had plenty of time to get things ready for us.

I worked my little Native butt off during the day, even walking to work and back. I was determined to get things done and prove to myself and to others that I could change my life path. I wanted my family at home in Eskasoni to be proud of me as well. I had a dream, a dream to get my book *Savaged to Wellness* published. I wanted to share my story with people. I wanted them to understand the process that happened and how it happened. I wanted to finish the end and submit my book to a publisher. So, I decided to start typing again, to finish what I had started at the women's center in prison when I was incarcerated for a year for a mistake that I must live with forever. I was about ten minutes away from the public library. I made a set weekly time to write to finish my manuscript. I was proud that I had written about ninety thousand words while serving my time.

I wanted to get my book published but had absolutely no clue what I was doing, no clue. I figured it out as I went, to be completely honest. I called a place and asked if they would be interested and for a slight fee that I could make my dream into a reality. It is a huge step to take on. Being in the public eye would be a little scary. Especially for someone like myself, an introverted addict/ alcoholic.

Insanity was me when I was running wild with my thoughts. I had some ideas of what my creation would look like, a book cover, and title. I did not even have a name for my book yet. I wanted it to be a Maine coastal cover with myself and my son. I was not sure. I reached out to as many people that I could that might be interested. I started making myself go to that public library to type and finish my book. I finally did receive a phone call from a publisher from North Carolina. I sent them my unfinished version. The ending was still absent, and I was afraid that I would not get it finished on time. With my entire busy schedule and everything else that I was trying to fit in. I finished the ending of *Savaged* in about seven weeks.

I sent my manuscript in to the publisher, then I received an email saying: "Melody, we are so excited to read your manuscript. We will let you know when we decide to publish or decline the book, thank you."

After a few weeks, I received a certified letter in the mail. I opened it and read it as quickly as I could. My heart was pounding with excitement. The letter stated, "Congratulations, Melody we are pleased to inform you that your manuscript has been accepted. Also, there was a three-page contract included. I knew that I would have to do my research, would need some legal advice as well.

It was very overwhelming as you could imagine. I did not know what I was doing. I was getting my "goals" in order and I was trying to figure things out at the same time. Nobody but my recovery people knew that I had a book coming out. I did announce it on my social media page that I would have a book "coming soon." I did not even have a title to the book yet. I was originally going to call it "Bits of Me," but I found out that name was already used. So, I started thinking of names for my memoir.

I thought about Wellness, Recovery, Moving on, etc. Took me months to get another name. I talked to Charlie about it and sometimes we joked on the phone about my savage ways. I would call him a beast and he would call me a savage, honesty not in a racial way just playing around. I do not take offence to the title "savage." It's a way I feel I use to be when I was acting foolishly when being a drunkard.

I suggested "Savaged and Well" He said, "No, that is not it. So, it took another few days, then one morning, I thought, *Well, I am recovering, and I feel well now*. I thought *Savaged to Wellness* will and could fit. I knew there would be some controversy surrounding this title. I was not afraid of it, nobody understands what I have been through, it hasn't been easy for me. I think that when I was living dangerously and carefree that was "Savage Mode" a beastie lifestyle living outside at times. It was not tame, that's for sure. Today I live to be free from all torments, including those that bind me in anyway. Binding my art form, writing is my form of art, yes, I am artist. So that is when I decided that I would use the name and I called my publishing assistant to inform her of my decision. It's not easy to make such "adult decisions." It's overwhelming at times to be "adulting."

Today I like the title *Savaged to Wellness*. It is mine. I own it, and if nobody likes it, well…that is their choice. I am not afraid of what others think of me anymore. I am free from all that drama today. I love my titles and I will not stop expressing myself.

I had a good friend of mine help me get access to a lawyer's office to read the contract over and make sure that everything was in proper order. I made sure I was prepared for everything because I knew deep down inside of me that my inner beast could be released again with life stressors. Such as lawsuits and other possible stressful situations. Today I like to try to not have any turmoil or drama because it is not for me. Then I was in the clear with my contract, I signed it and sent it back with the fee that was involved with it. Yes, I did self-publish and there are fees to everything including getting a book published to the world. I knew that I would make my family proud and make an enormous difference in how people looked at me. Could they understand me? I wrote my first book as an explanation to my madness. I wanted to apologize but also to explain a bit of my illness, my mental illness (ADDICTION) and recovery process. My process to wellness and self-knowledge of my illness and actions.

After a few days passed and I did not hear from Charlie, I thought he might have been thrown into the "hole" aka prison segregation. I was never in trouble when I was in prison because honestly, I stayed distant with everyone. Charlie told me that the men were sometimes challenging. It was difficult to sometimes work things out so there was a lot of physical fighting that would go on. That is how they settled things. I could not imagine the beastly behavior. I was worried about Charlie sometimes. I knew he had a temper and I've seen him get beastly at times. Then I received a phone call from him and yes sure enough he had been in "seg" of the prison. Charlie said to me, "Hi, babe, I wasn't able to call you because I was in 'Pods.'" I remember the pods as being dark and damp with no fresh air. The air was stale and suffocating. It felt like the walls were caving in. I did not enjoy the time when I was there in my fourth month of incarceration back in 2017.

Charlie explained to me that one of the "men" in the dorm was acting disrespectful to him and they were gesturing an inappropriate act. Charlie assaulted the man and almost hurt him badly. The way he explained it: "the mother sucker attempted to hit me; then I pushed him across the hall and that is when he hit his head. Almost knocking him out and lucky no injuries were reported as another charge." I told Charlie that people will push you but do not lose sight of what you're working towards. I mentioned to him that I had plans to help him get stable when he is free and that I would provide what he needs when he gets out. I felt good reassuring Charlie; he was my best friend and, although I was not sure where our relationship was going, I felt happy in my heart knowing that I could help another addict.

I stayed connected with Charlie, and I did make sure he always had money on his "books" as they like to call it in prison. His commissary was always loaded each week by me. I would make sure I would send what I could after I bought everything that I needed. The first few months of my incarceration I had no money, and nobody was sending me commissary money. To be truly honest, I did not care because I knew that being locked away was my punishment. I did not want to spoil myself in any way. I became extremely disciplined in prison.

I continued with my life, my routine, my meetings, my son, etc. Life was good, and I felt it would only get better. When I would sit in recovery meeting and people gave me a "who are you look," I would just smile. Slowly in my recovery meeting I started to open up, and I would share my weekly struggles and also, I would share my life. I was able to share that I was a writer and working on a book that I just needed a title and book cover. I had these big plans that were my recovery goals.

Charlie only had a few weeks until his sentence was up. During those weeks is when I purchased his clothes, hygiene products and a cell phone for him. During one of our nightly conversations Charlie asked me if I could get him the newest cell phone. I was kind of mad for a minute, then I remembered to breathe and remind myself that this was a moment that I had to say NO. I said to him: "Charlie, I'm very sorry, but you will get the same phone that I have, because it's what I can afford." It's a phone. I didn't have anything high tech. It was about two years older than the expensive phones, and I did not care as long as I could make and receive phone calls and look on the internet—then I was good.

I have never been high maintenance to be really honest. Since moving to Maine, I enjoy yard sales and I shop regularly at Goodwill. I would much rather buy clothes that are good brands but not with the price of some stores. I grew up having to pretend that my parents had money but, in all reality, they were poor. My parents were just getting by, feeding us, clothing us with sometimes labeled clothes as a present. I grew up with no cell phones and the only technology was the radio with limited stations. I could not understand why some of my friends even wanted me to be a part of their "cool group." I was poor and wore hand-me-downs.

I guess that's been with me now since I could remember. Material things became unimportant to me, so much so that I did not care if I had anything. Charlie grew up in a home where both his parents were hardworking farmers and worked outside the home as well. Luxuries were a regular to Charlie and his family. Growing up in a town in Maine called Fort Fairfield in Aroostook County. Charlie talked about the county and how nice it was growing up there in that countryside of Maine. Charlie talked about it regularly to me. I never really went up to that part of Maine, but I hear about it a lot. I hear that it is peaceful with lots of beautiful views; photos that I have seen prove it's nice. My friend Linda Theriault-Quirion takes these wonderful photos and posts them on social media.

When I was working, sometimes I would be able to pick up extra shifts at work to save more money. I had most all of my bills covered while working at the coffee shop and I had that weekly child support that I was paying. I had just enough to pay bills and place most of my extra spending to either Charlie or spend on my son. I did not care too much about eating at restaurants or shopping for fancy clothes. I'm a simple woman and I don't expect a lot. I'm very happy that I'm alive and just free from my disease. I like to remind myself on a regular basis of my clear mind, clean mind, calm mind.

Once the days became routine to me, I became a regular at most meetings and I slowly started to become comfortable with others. Slowly allowing others inside was a healing feeling. I was starting to open up to people in my recovery groups. I would just vent out if I were annoyed, overly emotional, lonely, and afraid…etc. I was starting to let the natural laws of life take over my soul. I was healing my damaged soul; I was recovering.

It was starting to get closer and closer to the date that Charlie would be freed from the prison walls. To be 100-percent-honest, I was terrified. I was afraid of relapsing with Charlie, I did not want anyone or anything to stress me enough that I would go into relapse mode again. I felt very anxious, afraid, worried, alone, angry at the thought of Charlie possibility triggering me to use the insane substance heroin again.

Heroin, the drug that kills and destroys lives, the drug that changes people into soulless human zombies. I once wrote an article that states "the zombie zone." I have seen and lived those hellish evil ways. These were the worst days of my life. When I was injecting *poison* into my human body, I became someone else altogether. This is when a person on substance will destroy everything in their path to just "get a high" that is like taking a substance that escapes a person from life.

It was Christmastime 2018 and I was alone, and I had just recently moved into a larger apartment down the hallway. Across the hall from me was a couple that I will call "Jay" and his wife, "Jill." They had a young daughter. She was about eight years old. One day while I came home, I overheard the couple in a heated argument about whose fault it was that they couldn't get money to get high. I was sad for the little girl. I could hear her in the background included in the argument. It reminded me of the way I use to be when high on "pills" back in 2008. I was coming home one day, and I bumped into the three in the hallway and introduced myself. I always started most convos in, "Hello, my name is Melody and I am in recovery." On this day when I introduced myself, I said, "Hello, I'm your new neighbor that moved from down the hall to this larger apartment because I have a son as well." I also included that I was in recovery.

They both looked confused, then Jay lifted his head and looked and me in the eyes and said, "Well it's nice to finally meet you, Melody." After about four months in the building, Jay laughed and said, "You're like a ghost, we never see you," lol. I answered back to him, "Yes well, I try to keep myself busy." I laugh with them. Jay looked at me. "Melody if you ever need anything I am right across the hall just knock."

Although I knew that the weeks were coming closer and closer until Charlie's release date. The daily chats made me secure in our relationship. About a week before Charlie was to be released from prison, I gave him a major lecture during one of our calls. I answered the phone politely, "Hi, Charlie… babieeee. How are you today?"

His regular reply was positive. "Hi, wifey, I'm doing good today." Sharing his regular daily check-in. "How about you?"

I replied with: "Well, honey, I'm very scared of next week because I'm afraid that once you're out that you will choose the drugs and women over us." And that was it, Charlie assured me that he was not about to use any substance that would cause him to lose me or his freedom. I said to him, "Charlie, I just want to live the way that I am living today, to be free from drugs and crazy.

I told Charlie, basically as they say on the street, "I schooled" him on the apartment building. He did not know that I wouldn't stick around the building during the day, mostly because of the possible temptation. Also, I chose to remain busy during the days because it was crucial to my recovery. I was like the rabbit in the building always in a hurry when I was entering or exiting that building on Ohio Street. I would regularly hear drug deals in the halls because I knew the "GAME," the game of either exchange of drugs or exchange of money to get drugs.

I was like a mother nesting; I was getting the apartment ready for Charlie. I had bought a new queen bedroom set. I made the apartment as comfortable as I could. I bought Charlie a phone exactly like mine. I had a computer donated to me so that I could finish my first book: *Savaged to Wellness*. The living room/kitchen was comfortable as I liked as well. I wanted to start a new life with Charlie and leave the old life and old ways behind us forever. Well, the final days until the "day" we reunited was a bit overwhelming, I knew that anything could happen. That there would be an adjustment period. Lucky for me I had the tools of a program that kept me on the right path and helped me to remain calm and strong. Also, I had recently started to see a substance abuse counselor, who I can call "Rich." I felt ready for any challenges that might come up. I knew that I would have to be selfish. To only focus on my recovery that I would not allow even Charlie, my best friend, my partner, to jeopardize my recovery process. I wanted and craved desperately for a clean and fresh start.

I talked to my sponsor, Ana, about my worries and she reassured me that it was perfectly okay to have these uneasy feelings about my future with Charlie. Ana's exact words to me were: "your recovery comes before anything or anyone." I thanked her. I knew deep down that Charlie was sick and tired. The sick and suffering lifestyle that we had created into a hurricane had to be behind us. This new life, a rebirth had to take place. I had already started to do what I needed to do for us to have a good start—recovery program, employment, home.

The last few days I had left waiting for Charlie had to be the most anxious days. It felt as though I had an upcoming court date. I had talked with my co-worker at the coffee shop about it for months now. Loretta would ask me daily, "How many more months, Miss Mel?" She knew because I told her most everything. I would reply, "Just a few months." Then it became a few weeks, then days. I was glowing and filled with excitement as each day passed. The night before his release date, he called at his normal time. Charlie said in a soft voice, "Hello, babies, do you still want me?" I replied back just as quick, "Don't be silly now, babe, I've only waited for this for twenty-two months." The last time I had a chance to just hold Charlie was that morning of April 17, 2017. The date we got arrested for "trafficking" was the strangest day.

I woke up and Charlie was starting to twitch because of the heroin withdraws we were both having. We didn't even lay together that last night because it was too uneasy to lay together because of withdrawal. I did not even offer him coffee or anything. We just woke up ugly together, hardly saying two words together. Except that I was driving down east to get money to get us high again. Sad but true, we hardly spoke to each other that morning and I rushed to leave. I said to him, "I will be back later this afternoon, okay?"

He said, "Okay, babe, I'm not going anyplace but here."

Then I left to get gas, I hardly had enough gas to get down there, but I didn't care. At my halfway mark, I had a strange feeling that I should turn back, but I didn't. Afterwards Charlie called me to tell me that he was arrested and that I should come home because I was being charged as well.

That had run through my mind while doing my time in prison for that year. When I would walk in the prison recreational area. I would see Charlie at when we were being held at the Knox County Jail. Then once or twice at Two Bridges County Jail. The morning I had court in Belfast for sentencing, Charlie was in the lobby. He had just been transported there and I was leaving for court. I knew that I had court, so I had a feeling I could see Charlie. I was escorted downstairs by the corrections officer. They gave me breakfast and a bagged lunch for court. The correctional officer said, "It's going to be a few minutes, Melody; we're waiting for transport." I said yes, okay, no worries. Then I heard the doors opening in the lobby, and I kid you not. There was Charlie in an orange jumpsuit. I recognized him right away from his height and build and that gray hair. I loved this man; he was my best friend. I thought about him hourly.

I yelled to him, "Charlie, hey Charlie it's me." He looked over at me. "Babieeee, hiii!" The guards told us to stop communicating. As I was being extra handcuffed for transport. I told Charlie, "I'm going to court and my lawyer said fifteen months. I will wait for you and write." He said, "Okay, babe. I'm looking at two to four years, but I'm going to fight it. Wait for me, Melody and write to me, okay?" I said okay. I looked over at him while I was exiting the building at Two Bridges and said to him, "I love you, Charlie." He replied back, "I love you, Mel." That was the last moment we had together in that lobby; after that we were both in prison where it's very secure.

The morning of Charlie's release date, I was so excited to see him. Just to have a real conversation with him without anyone watching us. It was going to be a fresh start for us. A chance to make things right with everyone we had caused any damage to. I was very determined to make this work and I was planning to do everything I could possibly do to help Charlie. Charlie came into my life for a reason. I feel that he helped me leave a relationship that was harming my soul. A relationship I stayed in for years just for my son.

I cleaned the apartment and I did everything that was asked of me. Food and Charlie's favorite snacks, all the supplies he would need like clothes, razors, toothbrush, etc.—it was all there. I had everything complete. I had even requested three days off, so I could spend time with him to adjust to the newness of everything. Honestly, it can be extremely overwhelming adjusting back to society. I remember my release date very well. I ended up drinking the day of. I looked for any excuse to get that cold beer down my dry throat. It was a sad moment for me.

I wanted Charlie to be stress free, to not worry about the small things that I didn't have. I was ready, I was all excited, I had even bought myself a special cute outfit. An outfit that I ended up not wearing that day. I wanted to be comfortable, so I just dressed in my favorite jeans and plain T-shirt. I called the taxicab to pick me up, and they arrived in less than five minutes as though the universe was helping me. Like a natural high that I was experiencing a natural adrenal rush, a happy moment was about to happen, and I was pumped. I jumped in the taxi, and I couldn't help but share my joy with this stranger. When I arrived at the bus station, I noticed there was not a bus yet. I was a bit relived. I felt for a moment that I wanted to throw up. I was able to just take a moment to say a prayer, a prayer for the both of us to like each other. We talked daily, we lived together before, and already knew each other. This time was very different, because we were both clean and sober from all substance. We did not have anything blocking our vision. I knew that there was a slight chance that I might not like Charlie, that he might not like me. That was the reality of our situation.

When I saw the bus pulling into the driveway at the bus station, I did not see him because of the dark tinted bus windows. As the doors open, I noticed a few people exit the bus. I noticed Charlie and he waved to me. Charlie still had his dark blue prison issued sweater and dark blue jeans on. I walked over and told him, "Welcome home, Charlie." He replied, "Thank you, Melody." We hugged each other for about two minutes and had a small kiss. It was a bit awkward; I had been so used to being alone that I felt like a virgin.

I told him that I already had a taxi waiting for us, but it hadn't arrived yet. He was all smiles; I took a few photos of us and that was it. Charlie said, "Hey, we have a taxi coming?" I said, "Yes, it should be here soon." I called the taxi company again, and they said, "It should be on the way." I noticed that Charlie seemed nervous. I looked over at him and said, "It's going to be fine, Charlie." The taxi driver pulled in. I helped Charlie with his bags. He had two large black garbage bags on him due to the fact that is what a person was given when leaving the prison. I felt bad for Charlie, I said to him, "We will get nicer luggage, okay?" He looked at me. "I'm just so happy to be free, honey. I don't care what I have."

When we arrived back at the apartment, it wasn't even noontime. Charlie looked at the building and I already knew what he was thinking. Charlie said to me, "We have to find a nicer building, babe." I replied back, "I know, but I made our apartment nice." We walked past the few apartment doors and went upstairs to the second floor. Mine was the first door on the left. I had cleaned the hallways that morning and sprayed air freshener. I had already talked to most of my neighbors about Charlie "getting out." When I opened the apartment door, the fresh smell of pine cleaner was still present.

I had cleaned the apartment the day before. There was cool chilly air coming from the kitchen window to air out some of the stale air. Charlie walked in and said, "Nice, you did an excellent job getting our home ready, thank you." I looked at him and smiled and enjoyed the moment. Charlie looked around and scoped out the whole place. Looked in the fridge and then asked if he could have something to eat. I said, "I can order Chinese food or pizza if you want." He looked over at me with a huge smile. "Really?" I replied, "Yes. We are not in Windham anymore, babe." I called the popular Chinese restaurant in our area and ordered Charlie some food. Basically, a small Chinese buffet was at our kitchen table and Charlie was all smiles. I did not want him to feel any pressure or added stress from his now new freedom. It can a bit overwhelming when being released from incarceration.

People that are just not aware can cause harm to a person as in trigger them to try to escape the reality or "numb out;" it's intense. I would advise anyone being released to have a support person for at least twenty-four hours. I was not so lucky, I lasted about two hours until I wanted to escape and just let loose. I ended up damaging a few relationships during this time. Today, I have had to make amends to the people that I used while getting drunk or high. Painful, but a hundred percent true that I am not fit to use substance. It changes every good in my body, mind, soul.

So, when Charlie was adjusting, I made sure that he had everything that he would need. I even had set up some services for him. I was able to get him in as a new patient, to see a substance abuse counselor. I was not going to have him violate his probation in any way. Charlie had like five years hanging over his head if he messed up in any way. I knew that I would not allow certain people that were using or triggers around him either. The only thing that I could not manage to fix as of yet was the apartment building. It could have been one of the worst buildings in Bangor, but it was still better than being out on the streets. That night Charlie and I cuddled up and watched some movies and just cuddled. I was happy just to have him beside me again with no guards around to tell us that we could not talk.

The next morning, I woke up early and left Charlie a note saying that I went to the gym to exercise. The working out daily was a part of my recovery program. As I was walking back early that morning from the gym, I noticed the moon still out. I was at the gym so early like they were open at four. I walked back slowly, and I remembered how we acted before our arrest.

We had acted like two crazed teens that had no clue how to live life. All we thought about was how to get high or find substance. I do believe that before our arrest, those were the darkest days of my life. I walked up the stairs. It was very quiet in the morning at our building. I was the only one awake and I could smell the coffee and I knew Charlie was awake. He was having a coffee at the kitchen table and said that he made me a cup. He asked me, "Did you have a good workout, babe?" I said to him with a smile, "Yes, babe." I sat there with him enjoying the moment and rugged coffee. It was nice having someone make me the cup of coffee. I felt the energy between us and this powerful connection like we had before the whole mess started. This connection with Charlie, I do believe that we are soul mates connected and reunited here on earth. Yes, as cheesy as that sounds.

I worked up the nerve to ask him if he would be interested in having some deep conversation with me. As in questions that were avoided due to our situation, like when we were apart. I wanted to wait for him to tell me what he thought I might have been doing while I was free from those prison walls. Charlie didn't know. If I was cheating or doing drugs secretly behind his back. Charlie gave me this strange look and said, "Melody, I honestly don't care what you did or didn't do, honey." He gave me this stare that I remember quite clearly. I didn't know how to react to that, so I just remained quiet as I stared back at him. That is when I knew that he was forgiving me for upsetting him at times, when I was drinking and answered his phone calls while highly under the influence of substance (drinking). I took it as a forgiveness and I was grateful and very thankful. Charlie then said, "You are here for me now and have helped me. Melody, you are my best friend and I love you very much, you have shown me that you are my woman."

The next few days, I started to realize that I had done right by standing beside Charlie. His life had a been crazy before he chose the recovery road. Charlie also had a dysfunctional childhood with what I can say as more traumatic than my own. I didn't realize it until later when I did my homework. Charlie's life is his to explain; I will leave it at that.

I also know that everyone makes mistakes that can be taken the wrong way due to abusive and dysfunctional families. But really who are we to be looking inside? When we are or haven't been invited. It's a path that I choose to stay away from because the past is gone forever, and the laws don't change.

Behind us is the insanity of substance use and abuse to our body. Today's date as I write this is July 4th, 2021, and this is a holiday. I will continue with the story.

I noticed that Charlie and I were getting along well. There were a few personal struggles. I would attend meetings and continued on my recovery journey. I felt a little bit more secure than before when we had been using heroin and acting foolish together. It was like a NEW relationship for us. We had not really been together clean or sober before. It was very scary for me; opening to anyone was uncomfortable for me. I was afraid and unsure how we would be able to grow together in our newfound recovery process.

Collaborating with a sponsor during my early months helped me in so many ways than one. I was able to call her when things became uncomfortable. I was able to look deeper than I have ever looked before at myself in the mirror. ACCEPTING myself as a damaged soul was when I started to really heal this angry inner child in me (core). I was able to calm myself down after knowing that forgiving myself for all the damage that I may have caused others during my life. This is where the spiritual awaking had happened for me. I knew then that I would be okay. The hardest thing that I had been brainwashed into thinking was that I was a no-good Indian that didn't deserve to be happy. Years of mentally abusive situations led me to believe that I would amount to nothing and that I was an ugly person.

That is a difficult pill to swallow, looking into the mirror and telling your-self you must let go and let God now. It is time to let go of all the hurt, pain, guilt, shame. Looking at myself back then and saying to myself: "Melody, you are a Native American woman who can overcome anything. Change your life path now before it is too late." Surrendering myself to my higher power, then letting go of old habits, old thinking, old ways. Rebirth, rebuild, relocate your-self with new people.

I also told Charlie that during our incarceration and this time apart from each other has healed me. I sat him down to tell him, "Charlie, I cannot deal with anyone that might jeopardize my recovery. So, if you're not serious, then don't bother me." Charlie took it well and with a glance at me, he said, "I com-pletely understand where you're coming from, Mel." He said, "I'm so happy that you have finally surrendered that lifestyle of drugs, alcohol, sex, trouble all around. Let's start fresh and allow this process to take place."

I continued working at the coffee shop, but I did want out, and wanted change. I needed healthcare and benefits that I deserved as a worker. That is when I knew that I needed to get a different job to fill this need. I decided that I would apply at one of the places that I worked before, way back before I had my son. Before my addictions took over my life and a place where I knew I could work the routine. I knew that this "company" would give me enough hours during the week and the benefits that I was looking for as well. I noticed one day during my internet time on social media that this "company" was hir-ing for a full-time position.

I applied for the job, then placed my resume with references as well. I mentioned that I was in recovery. I received a callback within a matter of hours. The general manager "Jim" was interested and wanted me to finish my appli-cation process as soon as possible. I was so excited about it that I told Charlie as soon as I could. First off, I said, "Hey, Charlie…so I filled out a job appli-cation at 'company.'" I said to him, "I have worked for them before, and they are a good company, and I would have benefits." Charlie looked confused at first then said, "Well, Melody if it is a job where you would have health care and benefits, then it seems like it's a good move." I was excited, I couldn't wait to finish my job application process.

The following day I received an email from Jim to inform me that if I was interested in getting started, I would have to get a drug screen first. To be honest with you, I had become use to having them weekly when I was at the prison, so it did not bother me one bit.

Although, I knew that I could and would pass the screen with nothing in my system, I was still a bit anxious about the situation. I knew that starting a new job with a new routine would be difficult for me. Just being newly recovered from my disease… well, I was scared.

Today, I'm in the beautiful city of Ellsworth, Maine. I'm sitting here typing this next book of mine. People are walking by and it's interesting to watch. This book business is not easy.

Anyways where was…. Oh yes starting a new job. I was asked to take the drug screen and I passed with excellence. I was to start my new job in just a couple of weeks. I wanted to give the coffee shop a decent two-week notice at least. I was trying to start a new path and leave my old ways behind me. One of the "old ways," "old habits" was leaving a job without notice. That was just mean and very irresponsible of me when I look back at it today. Back then it was just a part of my unmanageable lifestyle that I was leading. It was like when they say: "The blind, leading the blind." That was me. I wasn't too wise back then; I just didn't care about anyone. I did not care about anything but getting my own needs met. I was extremely sick and suffering when I was in my twenties. I remember working at a place for only an hour, then I walked off because I did not like the way the manager talked to me. It was just the insanity of the life I was leading at the time.

The next few weeks went by quickly and I was full of excited energy. I was so ready to leave the coffee shop behind me and start a different routine. I was ready to leave the old job behind me and I was ready to let the stress of it all go as well. On my first day at this "company," I was a bit nervous that I would meet people that I had worked with there before. I noticed that there were a few people that I noticed from local area recovery groups. Also, I did not notice anyone from before, so I felt a big relief. I mean so much time had already passed by, that I wasn't sure if I would remember them anyways. When it was time for me to start the workday, I was escorted to the hanging line by one of the supervisors.

I wasn't sure what to expect. I knew that I would be working with laundry. I was not sure which location I would be in this time around. I was placed in the linen, then shipping area last time when I worked for this company. The hanging line was a little different, I would be inspecting the uniform/clothes for missing buttons, holes in jeans, jean pockets, zippers and etc. I jumped right in to work mode. The hanging line consists of six people, who are inspecting and hanging shirts, jeans and uniforms. Inspecting clothes didn't seem too bad for a day's work. Not for me anyway. I was used to working doing about anything. I was not afraid to get my hands dirty, I enjoy work. Anything that would help me remain busy and pay my bills I was all for. This new job offered me benefits and a set schedule. It also gave me the security of having healthcare and dental care for the first time in years. I would be trained by a lady by the name of "Lori." Lori was one of these ladies that had been there for almost twenty years. She was a bit on the tough side at first. She would be working right behind me so in case I made any mistakes or needed help, she would be right there to help me. When I got set up to start work, I noticed that there was a bin full of jeans, a large blue bin with wheels on the bottom. A large bin that could hold a few hundred pounds of clothes. This one in particular had jeans, work jeans. I went and grabbed a pair then Lori showed me how to fold properly, so I followed her directions and I didn't complain about it. After a few hours, it was easy for me. It was working in a huge laundry mat. I did not mind working at this pace, especially after the stress of the other place before.

I was in a good place in my mind, I was happy about all the new things happening around me. My publisher was about to give me a release date for my upcoming "Savaged to wellness" book. I could not be more excited about it. My plan was to not tell anybody at my new job about authoring a book. I was there to work. I kept it a secret for the first few months. I just wanted to "fit in" with my new co-workers, I wanted them to get to know me first. I tried my absolute best to keep my regular life and my work life completely separate. After a few weeks I adjusted well at my new job, I even made a few friends. One of the ladies that I became close with quickly was tiffany, she was always there to help me when I needed it. Tiffany always treated me kindly and respectful. She became one my best friends at work in just a few short months.

Tiffany is the first person at work that I said that I had wrote a memoir about my recovery process. She was surprised about it at first. I was not sure if she might have thought I was crazy, making up stories. She is one of those happy go lucky girl that is hard to forget.

I really had never done anything like write a book before. It was something new to me, I did not even believe that I could actually finish this therapy of mine and make it into reality like I did. It all happened in like a flow like stage. Charlie was there with me every step of the way. He was getting ready to start working again himself but noticed that his hip was bothering him. I knew that it was a problem because he would talk to me about it when we would walk together.

I was afraid that if he were to get the surgery gone that it would increase his chances of being around pain medications again. This is where I had to sit him down and have a serious talk with him one day. I finished my first cup of coffee and walk, Charlie sat down with me. He said "Mel, I know you have every reason to be worried about having surgery," but I am telling you right now that I will not start using drugs again, I promise you. All I could think of was when he had to have surgery before. Trust and believe me when I say this that it was not ever good. I had only known Charlie for a few years but was with him during some of his surgeries and it always ended up with a relapse of substance…usually heroin.

That was my fear, which was the only drug I knew of that could send a person in such a major down cycle of destruction. It scared me in my core because this last relapse had taken us on this war path of self-sabotage that was what I like to call "zombie zone." Where a person gets completely obsessed with getting this high and would do anything to achieve this high. I glanced over to him, with this serious look. I said to him, "I do not want pain pills around me or in my home, Charlie. It's a gateway to getting high." Charlie looked at me with these sad eyes then replied to me instantly, "Melody, I'm trying to be a good man for you today. The last thing I want is to get high." I got to be honest, I was terrified of getting the crazed Charlie back into my life. I was profoundly serious about staying clean and leaving that old life behind. I pleaded with him for about a half hour, well our voices raised. I said to him "Charlie, I am afraid, I am afraid to lose you again, not just only to the walls of the prison but by overdose. It was all too familiar to me when I think back at our crazy active addiction lifestyle. We would act so insane while high on either heroin or cocaine…or anything to "numb us out." It was a life of sadness when I think back on it today. Living to "numb" is absolutely nothing that I am interested in anymore. Back then Charlie and I would not bother making dinner or breakfast, substance was our only thought. We hit food cupboards and lived off the government monthly "food card." It was once a week that we would have enough food to make a decent meal then sit down to eat together. I do not miss that life one bit.

Anyways, after talking about this hip surgery. We decided that it was something that would help his pain and get it so that he could start working part time again. He promised that he would stick to the lowest dose given to him for his pain management. I also had to prepare myself mentally in case something went wrong during or after his surgery. Before would be the easy part where I had to make sure I had a proper game plan in case something went wrong. He wanted a new hip and wanted to not be in pain, so I finally agreed that I would be supportive, just if he took the medications as prescribed by his doctors after the surgery.

This was an always scary road for me, medication management was something that I couldn't do myself. As an addict, I would take the double dose then worse…run out usually a week or two after my monthly prescription was filled. Then be out of meds for the rest of the month. After seeing Charlie abuse his medications before by sharing them with me but also taking too much at a time. It was a scary and challenging situation that I really did not want to face so new in my recovery time.

I wanted a new life with this man, I did not want the old crazy lifestyle we had before prison. I was ready to get well, and I needed someone as serious as me beside me as well. I knew that it would not be easy, I knew it would be a challenge.

The day of Charlies surgery, I had drove him over to the hospital. He looked extremely nervous and worried. I was also worried about him. I did not know if he would survive the ordeal of such a huge procedure. I mean really to "remove the old hip" cutting his bone just gave me the creeps. I was scared for him. Something told me that he would be okay though. Charlie was a tough man.

I had seen him in the hospital many times before. Before this he was in a Boston hospital recovering from Endocarditis. An infection of the hearts inner lining, usually involving the heart valves. The infection is treatable with IV antibiotics and usually a hospital stay. He spent his time in a place in a rehabilitation after care hospital in Peabody Massachusetts. He stayed there for about seven weeks, I traveled down there to visit him weekly or bi-weekly. It was difficult to see him hooked up to so many medical devices. The morning of the hip replacement, I had dropped him off that morning, then I went to work. I did this because its structure for me. Today I stick to the plan of my weekday and work around other things. Meetings, mom life, chores etc. He knew that I would be there when he was out of his procedure. A nurse called me right at exactly three thirty to let me know that he was all done and that he was in the recovering area. I did not mind going over to visit. Seriously I do not know why but I like to visit the hospital, I think its maybe because I feel safe. I am a Hypochondriac; it is a condition I've had ever since I could remember. I could not wait to see him; I was extremely excited and overwhelmed at the same time. I walked over to the nurse's station, there was a kind nurse already knew it was me. I was not sure if Charlie told him that I was native American or just that he described me.

I could hear Charlie charming the nurses. I could hear them laughing away like nothing serious was happening. I walked in and investigated Charlies eyes. I knew he was okay. With a big deep breath, I said to him, "Well, I'm so happy that your surgery was successful; I was so worried about that." He looked at me and said, "Mel, you know I'm not ready to leave you." We both smiled and hugged for a good two minutes. The hospital room was the very end of the hallway, so I knew what this meant, also they placed him in a room all by himself. I felt bad for him, so I stayed there for the night with him until morning. I woke him up, "Charlie, I must get to work now honey, I will be back afterwork again today." He was half-asleep, then just nodded to me with a smile. I rushed home to get my breakfast and coffee into me so that I could do my job. The day went by smoothly without any chaotic moments. I just tried my best to continue my work and lifestyle because that is what kept me accountable as an adult. So "Adulting" was new to me, I had spent some many years avoiding major commitments. Even things that I considered "weigh downs" was simple as a full-time employment.

I called my sponsor to check in with her about all this. I usually made it a weekly visit with her. Depending on the severity of my situation. This was considered a major issue, mostly because there would be Opioids in the home afterwards. I called her and told her that he a was in their recovery area in the hospital. She was a good support person for me when I needed just to calm down about things. I felt comfort in knowing that I could always call her for anything, even just advice. I went back to visit Charlie in the hospital. Only this time he seemed a bit "out of it" he had asked for some valium to "help his anxiety." I was so annoyed after he told me. I just shook my head because I knew that he did not need those for that. It was just another added drug mixed in with his "pain management." I sat down next to him I talked to him about my day, before I decided to railroad him with my thoughts. He looked over at me with a big smile then said, "Melody, what's the matter?" I looked at him with a serious look then said, "It bothers me that they have added valium to your medication list when it's a highly addictive pill." He just justified it by saying, "I could not sleep last night. I needed something to calm me." I knew it was not good especially considering his addict thinking. It is easy to get back into just "justify" a medication is clearly a red flag to me.

I knew that I had a storm brewing, but I was not exactly sure how I could prepare myself. I knew that any pills could be detrimental to my own recovery process. It scared me to my inner core. All I could think about was when I use to take multiple pills to ease any physical, emotional, and make up "pain" to numb me completely. A gateway to trouble of the mind, body, soul. I knew all about the troubles of what is known on the street as "benzos" could be capable of major damage. I used valium for years thinking I was easy in my anxiety. In all reality I was just trying to escape my reality which is sad. I do not believe I was in the healthy frame of mind for years. Six years to be exact that I was doing what I like to call the "pill shuffle."

I left the visit earlier than I would have if he wasn't so high on medications. Visiting Charlie that day caused me to have triggering thoughts. It was very close to home that it made me want to "escape" again. I decided to take the steps that I needed to continue my recovery road, which was to get my tiny native ass to a meeting, AS SOON AS POSSIBLE.

I had this heavy load to finish my first book. I had not yet completed the ending, I felt pressure about it. I could have easily lost it. I was so new to recovery, that I had to be alone just to be able to think clearly at times. My mind is not well because I'm an addict but also, I suffer with mental health issues such as ADHD with general anxiety disorder, post-traumatic stress disorder. Simple things I do struggle with, liked grocery stores, shopping malls. Its pains me to think how I over medicated myself for years without the proper doctor to help me.

The next morning, I went to work I tried my best to not face any thoughts about the possibility of a relapse. The thought of going down that dark path of pill use would lead me to drinking. I caught myself daydreaming a few times at work about substance. I wasn't really in the clear yet, I knew that I needed to put up my armor, in order to stay safe. Really the reality of my situation was bare skin like. It's not safe for an addict to be around any mind-altering substance. Our sick mind wants us to glorify the "high" so we fall into the zombie zone again.

After work I went back to the hospital to visit Charlie, once again he was asking the nurses for more medication. I was quite annoyed within the first few minutes. I said to Charlie in my most serious voice, "Charlie, you cannot have any valium because its highly addictive and you really don't need it." He looked at me with sad eyes, then said, "How do you know that I don't need it. You're not a doctor." That was typical of him to become defensive with me. My recovery was more important to me than anything. I made sure that he knew that. I left the visit early that day. Honestly, I felt slightly triggered watching him "nodding out." I knew that I needed to be with people that understood my struggle, so I went to a meeting that day.

A few days later, Charlie was discharged from the hospital. He had just had a hip replacement so naturally the hospital loaded him up with pain managing medication. I went to pick him up he was sitting there in a wheelchair at the waiting area of the hospital. He looked miserable; he tried his best to get in the car. While driving home he handed me a prescription for pain pills.

I read the note, it called for fifty Oxycodone five milligrams per table to take six tables daily. I drove to the local pharmacy to fill the order, honestly even that had triggered me a bit. The years I spent doing the pill shuffle I knew exactly what kind of danger was near. The mood swings, the craving, the detox. All of it I did for years without a rest. It brought me back to a dark place just this small task to fill some "meds."

When we arrived back to the apartment Charlie asked for his bottle of pills. I reminded him that over taking will just be a bad thing. He took what was prescribed for the first few days. Then the following days I noticed a slight change in his routine. His demeanor changed slightly in the following days. It's like he couldn't wait until I was gone to work. Charlie told me that he hid his bottle so that I wouldn't be tempted to use. I looked for his bottle of pills when he was showering and I found only five pills left from a whole weeks' worth, it had only been a few days, but I guess he was taking way more. Which doesn't surprise me one bit. He had overdosed several times on me before our arrest back in 2017. I didn't want Charlie to become addicted once again. I talked to him about the dangers road he was taking and really that's all I could do at that time. I looked the other way for a few days after. I noticed his withdrawal from the opioids for a few days. Once the day came where he was able to refill the bottle he was once again "up and around" doing un-necessary chores. I knew that I needed to figure out a way to help him but not cause damage to myself. It hit a boiling point when I caught him crushing up his pain medication one day when I returned from work.

I walked in one afternoon to catch him with a white substance on the table. I said to him, "Charlie, really? Why are you misusing your medications and jeopardizing my recovery as well?" He looked at me with this dumbfounded look and replied with "Because, I can't take what they prescribe, it's not enough. I looked at him then said, "Are you sure, Charlie? Do you know that this is the road to trouble and relapse?" We sat down to talk about it. I made sure to let him know that I can't be in a relationship with anyone that wasn't in recovery.

We came to a slight solution that I would be able to "hold his bottle of controlled narcotic" for him until he healed from the surgery. This was not a good solution, it placed me in a danger zone with my own recovery, but at the time I was still so new to the recovery process that I couldn't see this danger. A danger that could ultimately cause me to relapse as well. Not only was this illegal but also, I could get a charge for doing this, but I did it anyways. I thought that I could help but really, I was harming my recovery process. I carried this bottle with me in my glove compartment for a few weeks. Then I told him maybe its best if you start to detox yourself.

Charlie looked at me then said, "Okay, I can try it now that the pain has gone a bit." His hip wound was still there, but it was getting infected from the "ups and downs" of his…what I will call his pill bender. The wound area was red and puffy. I thought that he was just making it all up. But when he went to his doctor's appointment, the doctor placed him on an IV unit of antibiotics (basically another PICC line) I was totally panicked about this. Charlie had gone through this PICC line before, and I already knew that he placed heroin into a PICC line before. What is a PICC line? Okay to better explain. A peripherally inserted central catheter, less commonly called a percutaneous indwelling central catheter, is a form of intravenous access that can be used for a prolonged period of time or for administration of substances that should not be done peripherally.

That scared me, especially with all the known drug activity in our apartment building. It was something that I could not control. It honestly was something that I had to give to my Higher Power. I prayed about it, especially the fact that I could find him overdosed by his own doing. This was during COVID and everyone was doing a lot of stay at home "lockdown," this time that he had really not much to do. Once this PICC line was placed into his arm, Charlie made a promise that he wouldn't bother with it. He assured me that he didn't want to die this way. A few weeks passed by, and he seemed very serious, so I trusted him with his medication again. It would be his last few weeks.

But once again I found a container of white substance and asked him why and what he was doing. Charlie's answer was I wanted a better pain relief. I was angry and demanded that he stop the pain medication all together or he would have to find another place to live and that I wasn't going to stand for it.

I felt like my world was falling apart, I knew that I couldn't be with him once he started that old life once again. When I say "old life" I mean substance use and abuse.

I had another serious conversation with him. He agreed to stop the medication all together, this made me have some hope once more for our relationship. His opioid withdrawal was a few days, I think he handled it well, but it made me uncomfortable to watch him in such discomfort. A week of absence passed, then I started to see his change. Change to clarity and back to the road of sobriety. Then one morning I decided that I would be sneaky and check to see how he was doing.

I came home to Charlie earlier than usually to see if he was okay. I noticed Charlie acting strangely. By strangely what I mean is that he looked high. I could easily tell, especially if I have known someone for a while. You really can't try to con a con.

I demanded he come clean as to what he had placed into this PICC line. Charlie looked confused and surprised that I was even back from work so soon. Honestly when you're dealing with an addict you must get into a sneaky mindset as well. The old life to me is a disturbing one, an insanity that I really don't want to be a part of any longer. Sick world of destruction and possibly death.

I looked deep into his eyes as if I was trying to channel some demon of destruction. Then after a few moments, he admitted to me that it was Ritalin from the upstairs neighbors. The neighbors that were selling their medications. I was angry and very emotional, and I really didn't know what I was going to do…I said in my calmest voice, "Charlie, you need to stop this, or I will be forced to call your probation officer."

He looked at me with a serious face then said, "I'm sorry, Melody, I won't do it again, please." I said, "Serious this time?" He replied, "Yes, I don't want to go back to jail or die." I was just floored with anger that in my loudest voice so that really the neighbors could hear me. I yelled to him, "I refuse to live like this again, Charlie. You are buying drugs from fools isn't going to work for me." I walked back outside, then slammed the door on my way out.

I went for a walk to calm down, I could feel that my blood pressure was high. I had an overwhelming headache, and my face was red. I had had enough.

I was ready to call the probation officer, to place him under arrest, then returned to those dark prison walls of horror.

Once I calmed down a bit, I went back to check on him. I wanted to see if he was still alive and that he didn't have like a stroke or something. I opened the apartment door; Charlie was sitting at the kitchen table. He had a bag all packed. I asked him if he was leaving, he said to me, "Only if you want me to, Mel." I said to him, "Charlie, I don't want you to leave, but I need you to get serious now." Looking at him with this PICC line hanging from his arm, I told him, "Charlie, that's not meant to place random drugs into your blood, you could die. I don't really want you to die because you are my best friend and I really want you around."

Charlie sat down next to me, he gave me a hug then whispered "I love you melody, thank you for not giving up on me." We cried and had a serious conversation about our old life, how much damaged we had caused to ourselves and especially to others.

A few weeks had passed, the withdrawal, the discomfort, the agony had passed finally once again. Charlie seemed as though he was back to his sobriety mindset once again. I was so relieved, I felt as though my higher power was with us alone the way. I had a spiritual moment of peace that I was back on the road I needed. I wasn't going to just give up on him, like so many others did even his own family. The cruel words that I heard his own family speak about him was very heart breaking for me. I couldn't really understand why anyone could just "give up" on someone. In my culture natives stick beside one another no matter the situation, I mean if it's something that is forgivable. I can understand ones hurt pain and sorrow but really to hold a grudge until death seems wrong to me.

Once I stared to realized that I was back on my track of recovery I wanted to continue to work towards my goals again. Again, I didn't feel any distraction from my life. I started to re- edit my book, it took me a few weeks, just to be able to re write a lot of what I needed to correct. I decided to change almost every name in my first book, due to reasons of protection. It required a lot of skill and detail to re edit. It took me another few weeks to just be able to clean up the pages once again. It was ready to be resubmitted then finalized for publication. I was so excited, but I kept it a secret from my coworkers, I just didn't want anyone to make a big deal out of it. It was my journey and I wanted to share it with the world, and I was more than ready.

The publisher gave me one more final project. She wanted me to get a cover for the book. I had no problem with that whatsoever. But really, I had never published a book before. I had no clue what I was doing. I had hardly any help with these "Author" problems. My publishing assistance was very helpful when I had questions about anything. She had emailed me some ideas of some past book covers to give me some ideas.

I knew what I wanted; I wanted a coastal photo for my book cover. I wanted to show the coastal Maine waters. I couldn't afford a photographer. So, I started my research on some local photographers to see if they might have interest in photo credits. I made a few appointments, but they did not show up.

So, I decided to take it upon myself to finish "Savaged to wellness" my book. Really not knowing what I would get in return. I just desperately wanted it to be completed, I was ready.

One Sunday morning, like the Sunday morning today. When I was having a weekend visit with my son Anthony. I mentioned to him that I needed his help in finishing the book. That really, I needed his help in taking some photos of me for the book cover. I wasn't sure the destination of that day, but I did know where I was going…the coast. I took Anthony to breakfast that morning in Ellsworth my favorite town in Maine.

After breakfast we decided to drive to mount desert island, I especially love it in the fall when all the tourists have left, and it gets quiet. MDI is what most locals in the area call it—beautiful rocky shores with water views as clear as so tropical hot spots in the country. I love Maine that's why I choose to live here, all the local characters that come along with this magical spot. I was able to just pick a place that could catch all the beauty of the coast and have kind of an art theme. I drove to the bass harbor light house; I knew that I could possibly get some good shots there with the trees and ocean background. I had a vision, a vision of me sitting by the ocean looking into the waters… like the book cover was made.

I looked at the rocky shoreline; this is where I knew I needed to be. I asked Anthony to take as many photos as possible of me using my cell phone. Yes, I said it a cell phone photo that is the cover shot. I didn't know what I was doing. All I knew is that I needed to get a decent shot of me for my book cover.

Just like that after about a hundred or more different shots I knew I had the one that I would use. The one where I was sitting with a bit of a smile, looking into the sky and ocean, as if I was sitting there dreaming of what could be. There you have it, my secret to my first book cover.

After the long drive back, I drove my son back home to his father's where he was residing at the time. We had a good day with many adventures. I talked to Anthony about the photo credits already and I mentioned to him that his name would be used as photo credits. He was very pleased about this, I assured him that I would place his name on the cover.

That afternoon, I looked at all the different photos that were taken. I couldn't decide as to which one I would use. To me they all looked beautiful. The photo that especially got my attention was the one that I had imagined for months in my head. Me sitting alongside the coastal rocks, looking over to the east. I felt like it was the perfect photo to use as my book cover for "savaged to wellness" my memoir.

The next day after working at the coffee shop, I called my publishing assistant "Diane." I would usually call her whenever I had some news or updates or ideas about my book and the whole process. She always knew exactly what to say to me. I called her and said, "Hi, Diane, guess what? I could hear the excitement in her voice, she replied, what's up melody? Did you get your cover shot like you wanted?

I replied back, "Yes, I did and its beautiful." She said, "Send me the pictures so that we can start the photo editing part as soon as possible so that your book can be a book. Honestly after months of editing months of re-writing some names, re-writing the ending a bit. I was ready to summit the final manuscript. I was beside myself with excitement, I just couldn't believe that I would be the first in my family to become an Author. After causing some much harm and so much damage to everyone. I had a chance to show my people (Micmac's) that I can make you proud of me. I was just beside myself with joy and humbleness.

When I called my publishing assistant to talk more about my manuscript, Diane told me that it would take another six weeks to print and officially publish the book and get it in stores for sale. Diane said to me, "Melody, you have to make this book your full-time job. You have to give it all you got." I said to her, "Diane, I've been waiting for this book for months and I already have people wanting to order copies." I was very anxious about the book, and I didn't know anything about this new world of "Author Life." I told her, "I understand everything takes time, so I will take a step back and trust this process." I still don't know as much as I would like about the world of books.

Well, after waiting patiently I noticed an email from my publishing company. When I went to open it, it read…Congratulations, Melody Paul, on your new book, titled *Savaged to Wellness* set for distribution in March 2020. I was so excited to share the news with everyone that was supporting me in my recovery as well as my life. I placed a copy of the book cover on one of my social media pages which read…. My upcoming memoir coming soon to book stores near you.

The post blew up with support especially from back home in Eskasoni, which made me so happy. When I shamed my community was back in 2017, when I was arrested for trafficking, and everyone was saying very negative things about me. I heard this from people on my social media pages and from my own family. That I was a disgrace to my people, a disgrace to my family. That really hurt my inner core, it caused me a lot of sleepless nights while I served the time in prison. Those painful words made me think about what I had made of my life up to that point thought. I thought about the hurtful gossip that was going around about me that I intentionally caused someone's death and that I was a murder…. That especially hurt me.

Well, the fact of the matter is, I did give an unwell addict a substance that unfortunately took her life. Which was ruled a result of an overdose on substance. I myself was in a very sick state of mind because I was in my down world spiral of active addiction, bottom line I wasn't me. People don't understand the "junkie addict" that asks for change on streetcorners, or the hookers that walk to sell their body for the next fix. It's a disease of addiction that makes people do horrible self-harm to themselves because they have no help. This reality of my today is that I do understand my addict a bit more. I understand that when I was sick, I would do the most insane and disgraceful things, just to get the "high." The high that only lasted a few moments, moments enough to numb out any emotional pain I was feeling. I didn't want to hurt anymore. Pain is what causes us to harm ourselves and others.

Today I don't have to feel this pain because I choose this recovery.

Where was I…? Oh yes, my community support and hometown joy. People commented positive things on that one social media post. I was so happy, and I didn't know what else to do but to thank my creator once more. For helping me to see what I needed to see before it was too late.

I received messages about orders, messages of hope, messages of love, and yes, some inappropriate messages that I had to either block or ignore. Yes, I was on my way to having a book., something I could be proud of. Finally, after years of killing my inner core with self-sabotage I would have a "title" like my sister Trudy has the Rn. I would have "Author "Melody Paul, how exciting. I knew this new road I was traveling, this new world of RECOVERY. Letting go of the old me and moving forward with a new lifestyle that I was creating.

The first person to hear me say my book was Charlie, he was always right there to help me along with emotional support. I wasn't sure which direction everything would go. I didn't really know what I was doing. I didn't really know what was coming either. I knew that I had to keep on with everything else. I couldn't just quit my job that was paying all my bills to pursue this writing dream of mine.

I had so many thoughts running through my mind, I didn't know what to expect. I didn't even know where to start, I had no clue as to what I was doing. All I knew was that I would be able to make this book into reality and I was excited. During my journey, when I first started to write the pages of the memoir. I wasn't sure I could make it possible. Imagine sitting around in a county jail for hours with nothing to do. Yes, you must do something with this valuable time or get extremely bored.

The Knox County jail, the place I stayed for three months before being sent to prison, is where it all started for me with the book idea. This county jail had programs and self-help classes to help the inmates. So, I signed up for "school," a GED or hi-set as they called it today. I was introduced to Mike L, a teacher that had recently retired from the Maine correctional center as the teacher for the inmates at the Maine prison. Mike had this cool energy this Eric Clapton look and style. He used kind words with me and was very assertive as well. He would be direct and on point with me. I asked him a question, there would be no sugar coating. Mike was exactly the type of personality that reminded me of my school days back home in Eskasoni.

With some wise and very encouraging words from the hi-set teacher Mike. For one afternoon while I was studying, I noticed a local "free press paper." I read a few of the articles in this paper is when I noticed an article that caught my eye. This one recovery story where a woman was sharing her experience, strength, hope.

I talked to Mike about writing a statement about my recovery process and what I had done, the reason for my incarceration. I said to Mike, "I can do an article, I can write as well," Mike looked at me with this serious look, then replied, "Melody you can do anything you put your mind to." He believed in me and that is really what drove me to spend my time writing. I started the article off as when addicts are in the zombie zone, when they are so sick due to the disease of addiction is when they don't care who they hurt. After finishing this article "Zombie zone," I asked Mike if he could reach out to the paper to help me publish it. After a couple weeks of waiting for an answer…during one of my hi set classes, Mike was excited to tell me that he had "news." I wasn't exactly sure what he meant but all I know is that when you spend most of your day locked up in a room the size of a large apartment locked up with woman talking about things that weren't pleasant to hear, any news is refreshing.

When I sat down in the classroom, Mike said, "Melody, so I did receive word that the paper "free press" is very interested in publishing your article." I looked at him with excitement. The type of excitement a person gets when getting gifts at Christmastime. I had a natural adrenal rush, I answered back, "Awesome news." He mentioned that a woman by the name of "Patrisha Mclean" was interested in coming directly to the jail to interview me. I knew the name because she was a photojournalist and a well-known author in Maine. I couldn't believe how everything happened so instantaneously. There were still so many questions that I had about my life, like where exactly I was going and what I was to do when I left the jail. Honestly, if I even left. This ray of sunshine and hope Patrisha was bringing to my heart would be life-changing to me.

I was so ecstatic about this interview, I told everyone in the jail about it. The sergeant of the jail even had a talk with me about the positive and powerful impact it would bring, not only to the jail but with the inmates as well… the sergeant was so proud of me that she had me speaking at an event on the jails recent added on programs such as the meeting they would have that were recovery based.

When the day came for the interview, I made sure that I would be presentable to this newspaper, and I wanted to make a good first impression to Patrisha.

I ended up wearing my regular yellow jumpsuit, the one that the jail gives to all the inmates. I was personally very excited about meeting and talking with Patrisha. I sat down in the jail classroom just like it was an ordinary day in the classroom. I could tell how excited Mike was with just the energy that he brought into the room that day. He was smiling from ear to ear, than said to me, "I'm so proud of you" look at the impact you're going to have on this jail, just by sharing your recovery story. At the time I didn't really understand what that meant but today I do understand.

When Patrisha Mclean walked into the room, she had this spirit about her, that could overtake any room, the energy of a free spirit. The refreshing energy I felt from her was a relief from all the toxic energy I had felt from the other inmates. I was very refreshing and energized me to my core. She had this big, beautiful Hollywood smile. She glanced over at me and introduced herself, "Hi, Melody. It's a pleasure to meet you. I especially enjoyed the article you wrote for us for the paper." I was so honored, and I felt like a human again, honestly that interview made me believe that I could push myself to become someone. When the interview started it was a sit-down conversation between two artists. I had this sense of normal for as long as this interview lasted. Talking about how I came to be in this county jail to my plans where for the future. To be honest I had no plans at the time, I was a lost soul before I discovered writing and recovery. This interview seems to move me forward on a path of healing and inspired me to take my life seriously. I was able to see hope that I could change. Change for the better and possibly help others along this path. After about sixty-five minutes, the interview was over and there I was sitting, waiting to be escorted back to my cell. This is when Patrisha asked if she could take a tour of the jail and possibly get some ideas for a photo.

So, we both were escorted around the jail to take photos. Then ended up in the gym area where the inmates would practice their basketball skills.

The hand painted mural was done a few years back, it was a coastal shoreline. Patrisha said, "Let's take some photo right here," I just posed and smiled with the best of intentions. When the interview was over, she asked me if there was anything that she could do for me. I just answered her back, "Just a few of the photos and article when its printed would be nice," she smiled and said, "I can do that," I thanked her again, asked her for a hug. It was very nice during such a difficult time in my life. Today I'm proud to call her my friend, Patrisha was able to give me hope when I thought my life was over. Inspired me to move forward and push towards my goals. She is one of the people that I admire and look up to.

After that first article for *Maine Free Press*, it built just that little bit of confidence that I needed to push me to move forward. I wrote the "Zombie Zone of Drugs."

When the article was ready for publication after help with editing some areas of English that I needed help with it came out with that photo we had taken of the mural in the background. I felt as though I could accomplish anything, this natural high of adrenal I felt once again. It was from normal life experiences; it was from a pill or drink. It was natural high from doing something for my community.

A few weeks after I sent my final approval to my publisher, I received a phone call from Diane. I reached to answer my phone with excitement. I heard her voice. "Melody, the book is ready, we will be sending you five copies in a few weeks" I replied with excited voice, "really.... Awesome, thank you so much." Diane said to me," Melody you should be so proud of yourself for what you have done, is not easy to write a book." I thanked her once more, and then she said to me, "*Savaged to Wellness* will have a release date of March 8, 2020."

It was just the beginning of February, so I knew that I could take some down time until the book came out. After all I thought that I would be doing book signings and a mini tour around the tri states and Maritime provinces.

Although I knew that I might have to take on my book duties on a full-time basis, I wanted to give it all I had. I planned to take some time off from work to promote 'Savaged to wellness" By the end of February the news started to talk about a certain new virus overseas. A Virus that was causing massive hospitalization, a virus that nobody had ever heard about with no name. At the time I didn't think nothing of it, I thought it would be a virus like bird flu or chicken pox. Something that would just come…then leave us. As the weeks leading up to the book release came near is when slowly the numbers of people in the us were getting infected with the virus, this virus now had a name…COVID-19.

This was something new, even doctors didn't know anything about COVID. That was the scary part, an illness that caused illness so severe that it could cause death. Everyone in my area was in a panic. People started wearing masks in my area of the state. Then we were required to wear mask to work and have our temperature taken before we could clock in to work. It slowly became a shut down. Then once we started getting cases of COVID in my area of Bangor Maine everything would slowly either close completely or have certain times of the day for shopping. It felt like an end of the world horror movie. When doctors have a hard time to explain COVID, is when I became a bit nervous. Actually, not nervous, just scared to die really.

I already had a terrible disease, a disease that kills hundreds daily, a substance uses disorder disease. I knew that my disease had the potential to kill me if I didn't get my program of recovery in order daily. This new virus was causing so many deaths by late February that they shut down our state, then everything was shut down. Certain times of the day I went grocery shopping, which was early morning on Saturdays on my days off. I would get what I needed for us for the week, then go straight home, shut the door in the apartment building, then isolate with Charlie for the rest of the day. We watched a lot of movies during this time.

I was also given a note from work to show if I were to get pulled over from work. Nobody was allowed to be outside roaming around for no reason in

Bangor. This COVID virus was very contagious, it would spread from person to person like the common cold but with deadly symptoms. I wore a mask every place I went, even when I went to check my mail in my apartment building. This apartment building had homeless people using substance in the hallways and people would be injecting themselves with drugs as I walked by them. The apartment building had random homeless people also bunked in the downstairs hallways sleeping or passed out. Bottom line the building was dangerous in every way imaginable. I was very scared I would either get COVID or relapse during this time.

On March 8, 2020, I went to work as usual, then went straight home after. This time when I got home, Charlie looked at me than said, "You have a package here from your publisher." I looked at him, then got excited. "I think it's my book." I opened the box, which was about twenty pounds as fast as I could. This is when I saw the blue color of the front of the book, the ocean background photo that we took months before. I had my book in my hand; then I cried for joy. Charlie said to me, "This is a big deal, Mel, not everyone has a book." The first words out of my mouth were let's take video and photos. Charlie recorded me opening the box. Then with a big smile, I took a few photos. Then posted on the social media sites that my first batch of books had arrived. Honestly, I was planning to keep these copies for myself.

So many people from back home wanted details on how they could get a book. I was so honored to have people be so supportive, it was a bit over whelming. So, I decided that I would sell these copies that I had. I ordered forty books at first to see how many I could sell in my area. I sold out in a matter of days. I couldn't believe it, but still it was a scary time for everyone. It was right in the middle of COVID, there was precautions that I was taken. I made sure that I socially distance myself with my customers when there was a sale. After a couple weeks went by, I decided I would try my best to reach out to try to market my book. Everyone was either not in office or the business was completely closed due to COVID.

I felt stuck, I felt as though I worked so hard to be able to become a published Author that I didn't want to fail and fall on my face. I had no choice at the time, I couldn't do anything that I wanted but I did make the best of it. I sold books to people in my area, people back home were either ordering on Amazon or dealing directly with me.

My sister Trudy was helping me sell books back home in Cape Breton. She worked as a full-time nurse during the day; then after she was taking orders for me. She did very well and helped me break even with my investment. What made me so happy to my core was the fact that I made my family proud, also my community of Eskasoni proud as well. After all those negative comments and rumors went around my reservation back home, I was hurt and felt like I had caused shame to my people and especially to my family. This is another reason I wanted to write my story. So that people could understand a bit of the darkness what the addict goes through. Sometimes it could be your neighbor, your coworker, your family member …you just don't know. It's a very hard disease to have, it's also hard to get on the right path without some serious work.

Writing helped me in so many ways. I wanted them to understand my illness, my substance use disorder. Mostly I wanted to tell my side, my disease led me to do some really sick and unforgivable things but really, I was only human, a sick human. During COVID I noticed that most of the places that done meetings were closed. Honestly don't you remember how scare the world was during this time. We couldn't escape it.

I needed to continue my recovery twelve step program, so I reached out to friends in the program that were doing online meetings. I didn't know what zooming was. All I knew is that I hadn't attended a regular weekly meeting because they were all closed to public due to the COVID virus. It took me a while to get warmed up to online Zoom meetings. At first, I thought, that it wasn't personal, but once I tried the meeting, I was able to share my thoughts and the struggles I was going through. It wasn't so bad. I was able to be heard from my fellow addicts in these meetings, and that's all that mattered.

Pretty soon I was facilitating my own Zoom meeting, the weekly Wellbriety meeting normally held at the recovery center in Brewer. I had a group of recovery friends that needed a Thursday person to do a meeting, so I volunteered my time to help the community. Volunteering time is especially important when a person is in recovery. During our time in active addiction, we spent a lot of our time sucking the life out of everyone around us. To selfish to even know what we were doing besides the obvious. Soul sucking is what I like to call it. When we give our time to help others while in recovery, it really does help. During the "shut down" time I was able to focus on some things that I wanted to get done like this book that I'm currently working on.

Our local area had some meeting locations as well, places where people were meeting to talk or mini meetings. I would call sober friends and reach out to people that too were struggling with the beast of addiction. I turned my whole life into a process of healing my body mind and soul. Recovering from this substance use disorder was especially difficult for me during the pandemic. The time that I was scared to even step outside my "door yard" as some Mainers like to call the area of the adjacent to the most used door exciting the home where you live. I was scared to even go get my mail during certain parts of the day when there would be homeless people using drugs in the hallways.

It was so hard when I had to pick up the dirty needles that they left behind, they didn't have a care in the world. I once was there, I was once in that mental state., I knew to just let them be when they were injecting themselves with poison.

I can tell you this that during the pandemic, I was living in one of Bangor's roughest apartment buildings. Not only was it as nastiest as you can imagine on the outside, but the inside had a few apartments that were dealing drugs. I was torn in this strange cycle of COVID pandemic and living in these crazy building with so much drug activity. It's really a miracle that I didn't resort to giving into my demons during this time.

At about the time of COVID is when I started to make a name for myself with my book. I had no clue as to what to expect with this. My new reality was also dealing with my neighbors and with the pure insanity of my apartment building. A few times a month the traffic in the building was especially busy, this is when I knew the couple that lived upstairs from us would get their monthly medications. The hallways were full of people either nodding off or just looking like the wanted to grab whatever you had on you. Luckily for me I already knew how to approach them. Just walking past, with a smile is what I had to do… I had no choice because I didn't want trouble. When they asked me if I needed anything I would just say, "I'm good, I'm in recovery and I don't do anything today." I really don't know what was harder on me, the pandemic or the apartment building that I was living at.

I had to kick people out of the hallways for sleeping or call law enforcement on them a few times just so I could be a peace in my own apartment. That was a daily struggle when I was there at that Ohio street apartment. It was a nightmare living there. I didn't leave because the landlord had given me a chance and I was on a budget.

About mid-April 2020, I was struggling with just keeping on my own path of happiness, due to the fact that I hadn't been to a regular recovery group in weeks, I started to have thoughts of secretly drinking after work. I had thoughts of using drugs and going on a major bender once more. I was my own worst enemy really. I knew that my disease was trying to talk to me about feeding this demon. My whole thought process started to deteriorate, just because I wasn't getting any of my "recovery meetings." I finally decided to zoom a recovery meeting. I will be honest with you right now I didn't like it one bit. It was weird to me to call into a Zoom, then have people there in small boxes on the screen. It was hard for me to hear the other people speaking or talking over each other. I didn't want any part of it.

This was one month into the world crisis. It was pure insanity for me. I was thinking that I was going to try anything that would help me. I was totally desperate to get any kind of relief. I called my sponsor, Ana, and I asked her what I was thinking. The phone rang a few rings before she picked up. "Hello, Ana. How are you today?" Her response was always calming to me. "Hello, my dear friend. I'm doing as good as expected considering these circumstances. I took a deep breath, and I could hear she did as well. We stayed silent for a moment…. Then I said to her, "I'm struggling, and I am afraid that I might use or drink today." I was being honest with her. I had not felt so horrible (mentally) since I was in prison. She replied, "Melody, you are a strong, independent woman of worth and you don't need a drink or drug to feel better." For some reason just hearing her speak these words to me, it's when the words "sank in my head."

The thoughts of when I used to use came crashing into my mind. Horrible thoughts like waking up with the tremors and desperately looking for a drink so I could just feel better. Also, thoughts of when I was injecting myself with what I thought was heroin but was probably "mixed drugs" from random dealers, poison really. Imagine being so desperate to feel better that you would experiment with anything that looked as they would say on the street "Legit." This is when I came to the truth of my sickness. My powerlessness was clear.

The cold hard truth was that for me drinking or drugging would cause me harm and possibly death. I had started this new life without substance, and I was getting my life in order and manageable. I knew that if I went back out it would be trouble. After talking with Ana for a little over an hour, I said to her, "Ana, thank you for reminding me that I don't have to drink or drug today." She replied back, "It's what we do, my friend." I felt like I had the demon off my back removed. I knew that if I didn't keep a close eye on my disease of substance use in check that it could be deadly for me.

When I found that daily praying would help guide my sick thoughts elsewhere, maybe I was just piling my demon thoughts away. This is when I knew, I must talk to people when I'm upset. Letting go and trashing the thoughts instead of piling them like leaves in the backyard could be toxic. Toxic thoughts would lead me to death.

I started to read my recovery literature more often, I wanted the words from these books to sink into my mind like a memory. When I started to accept the fact that I wasn't normal is when I started to calm my mind. I had to get the information to these Zoom meetings and participate or else I could die from my disease. I know that today as I write this book. It was pretty much do or die.

During COVID everything was different. I started this routine of getting my groceries early in the morning during the days off from work. I would go when the doors would open usually around seven am. I would get supplies for the week for meals and supplies for the home. During the weekends I also started to walk what I like to call the "hills" in downtown Bangor. Bangor has a few steep hills. If you have ever visited Bangor, then you must know which hills that I'm talking about. State street, Park Street, York Street were especially good for me staying the weight that I wanted. The gym that I went daily was closed due to the pandemic. I had to maintain my exercise goals as much as my recovery goals. It was a daily routine for me to walk early in the mornings sometimes even before the sunrise. I had to pretty much step over the homeless people sleeping in the hallways of my building. Also, there was times I would literally catch people right as they injected the drugs in the hallways of the apartment building, I was living at. It would remind me of where I use to be. I would feel so bad for this fellow addict that had no clue that there was an actual solution to the madness.

Honestly, I knew from my experience that what they were doing was just trying to feel better. I would walk for about forty-five minutes before returning. Usually when I came back from my walk is when all the halls would clear out. This was the only time when this building didn't have random people. The Police were a regular presence at that apartment building. It was defiantly a daily challenge to live there.

When I went to work was my only escape from this nightmare apartment building.

My job was considered "essential work" washing uniforms for hospital workers was one of our new accounts, I noticed medical jackets also lab coats. Sometimes we would find old COVID test from the uniforms from the hospitals. It was especially hard when there was used needles found in the pockets of the lab coats. I didn't know at the time that I would be one of the lucky ones that wasn't "laid off" like most of the county, it was lifeline this job during the pandemic. Going to work during COVID helped me stay out of trouble. Unfortunately, they did lay off about twenty people, I was so relieved that I wasn't one of the people. I noticed one day they had gathered each in a group, then were given the bad news. It was such a sad thing to experience when coworkers were asked to leave to shorten the staff. I was extremely lucky that I wasn't one of those people. Being an addict, I wouldn't last too long in the community without something to do and something to actually look forward to. Working became my daily escape, not only for my soul but for my sanity as well.

I continued to work my regular program and my regular routine. Which included going to exercise daily. I knew that if I skipped even just one day that it could have a negative impact on my weight and also my mental health. Taking care of me was what I became focused on, my twelve-step program was also one of my daily goals. COVID caused many people in my area to pass away of complications from substance use disorder.

I had a friend of mine from the program reach out to me to let me know that I could facilitate a weekly Wellbriety meeting via Zoom. I knew it wouldn't be the same but at least there would be a meeting a gathering of the sick minds to help each other cope and talk about our disease of addiction. The facts were that either we would have to come together safely without complications like relapse or death. The Zoom meetings were new to everyone, nobody knew what to expect. People sometimes had a hard time even to log into a meeting because it was so new. But the reality of that time was that we needed to isolate at home in case one of us were to get COVID. Nobody knew what this COVID was about to cause massive world isolation.

The Zoom meetings were saving lives, the addicted person needs support daily to live an honest program. We need time to talk about our disease and the many symptoms of our sickness needs to be heard and support from our meetings, that is our medicine.

Once I practiced a few times how to log in and out of other Zoom meetings I was able to figure out what I needed to do to get my meeting going on a regular basis. I know that it sound strange to many people that support from meetings is a lifeline, but it truly is. When you wake up with the cold hard reality that you are an addict and willing to go to any length to get help to just live a normal life, then you will be ready to move forward. Sometimes people must fall many times to be able to see the light.

During one of my meetings, I was finally able to talk like at a regular twelve step meeting. I opened about my disease to my fellow addict, I spoke about my issues without worry and I was able to let go again. It brought me peace in my heart and ease to my inner core. Being an addict, especially one that is addicted to pretty much everything that feels good to me. I had a solution to my madness again, that solution was support from my fellow addict. Having people to share my struggles with has been instrumental in my recovery process. I've been able to heal my sickness with community rather than resorting to my old habits like the bottle or bottle of pills.

If you are reading this and are new in the program, please don't give up on yourself so easily. Life gets better especially if you work for it, work with a sponsor and do the work of the program, unity as in volunteer work. I was able to volunteer for my community the first year. It brought me to a humble space during that first year. To work somewhere as a service to the community was maybe one of the best things I could have ever done for my soul. I hope to volunteer my time again in the future, just because it brings good to my heart.

Anyway, back to the hell of living in the building on Ohio street during COVID. Once I was walking by one of my nicer neighbors "Sonny" he was about in his mid-fifties with a polite and good way about him. Sonny said to me, "Melody, my son is moving in with me temporarily until he can get back on his feet, his name is "jack." I always talked good with sonny during our conversations about the building or neighborhood. I said to sonny okay I will say hi to jack when I see him. One early morning I happen to meet him sitting near the steps beside his father's apartment door. I said to him, "Hi, Jack, my name is Melody. I live upstairs." He looked and smiled at me then replied, "Oh yes, he mentioned you." Me and Sonny were the only people in this drug-infested building that worked full-time jobs. One of the first things I told Jake was that I was in recovery and that I don't party at all. He looked at me with this strange look and said, "Oh, I see," then said, "I respect that girl." So that's when we came to our mutual understanding, I feel this to be true in my heart anyways.

Jack was very handsome man; he looks a bit like the actor from venom. Nice street way about him, he always was very polite to me when I passed him in the hallway. Either when I was on my way to work or just passing by. He was always there like some security guard for the building, but he wasn't. He was usually talking with the random homeless sleeping or using drugs in the hallways. For someone like myself in early recovery, it was extremely challenging for me to just enter and exit my apartment. Jack never really bothered me much thought, we would have conversations about life and how crazy it was at times. Jack wasn't in recovery, but he knew that there was a better way.

One evening as I was settling after dinner, I heard a loud scream from my bedroom. Which just so happens to be directly below Sonny and Jack's apartment. I heard sonny yelling "Jack, wake up" then again "Jack, wake up." I looked over to Charlie and said to him, "Jack needs Narcan, he must be over-dosing." I sat up from my bed and went over to my purse where I knew I had some Narcan spray. My heart was beating so fast when both me and Charlie ran down the hallway, then down the stairs. Knocked on their door like in a panic. It took a couple minutes for Sonny to come to the door. When the door open, we looked over to Sonny. He had almost a pale face with sweat running down the side. Sonny said, "He's not waking up, he's not responding to me, I don't know what he took today." I knew that Jack was using heroin sometimes, I knew because I was able to see my old self in him at times. I recognized when he was sober and when he was high just by his demeanor. When he was sitting in the halls in the building stairs drooling on himself was especially telling.

Sonny was so distraught and confused looking. I said to him, "Where is he, Sonny?" Sonny looked over to me with these desperate eyes, then said, "He's in my bathroom." I asked him if I could come in, he immediately said, "Yes, Melody, please." We walked in the apartment then sonny pointed the way to his bedroom. One look at him is all it took; I knew by the way he was slouched over on the toilet that he had been using. The blood from his needle injection was seeping down his arm. I looked at sonny and shook my head then said, "Sonny he needs this spray. It could bring him out of this and save his life." He gave us permission. Charlie slapped his cheeks a few times "Jack" wake up but no response. I said to Charlie use the Narcan. I had already used the Narcan before on Charlie three times, I knew it was what would bring jack back.

I opened the Narcan package as I was practically running down the hall, it was already open and ready for use. Charlie said to me, "Mel, how do I do it?" I said, "All you do is spray it directly into his nose." Charlie looked con-fused but followed my direction well. I looked at Sonny, then said to him, "I have had to do this before, so he will be a bit agitated when he wakes up. The three of us lay Jack on his father's bed. He started to breathe again. Jack opened his eyes; he honestly did look like that actor, and it reminded me of when he was freaking out in that restaurant when he took a bite of the live lobster. Jack shook his head, then sat up. "What's going on here? What happened?" Then I said, "You had a close call is what happened." He knew that we just saved his life, then the police arrived. I told the officers that we had some Narcan then gave him some. I gave a brief statement.

Jack and his father both hugged and thanked us. I said to Jack, "It doesn't have to be this way brother, there is a way." I wanted the police to take him away that night, but they didn't. The police presence was so regular at this building that nobody really got arrested, it was just like when I was in jail and the guards calmed a situation down. My heart hurt a bit for both. It's so hard when a person is in active addiction, but they decided to do the same pattern daily.

I won't sit here and write that this didn't faze me, that would be a lie. It bothered me to my inner core. It took me back to when I was actively injecting poisons into my body. I remembered when Charlie was laying on the floor unconscious then turning gray on me, yes gray. The first time I seen someone overdose was when I first started experimenting with heroin in 2016 before my incarceration.

I wasn't injecting anything yet, I was mostly vacuuming it up my nose, which is very gross. I had just started dating Charlie and I had no clue as to what this nasty disease could do to a person. I was already sick in my mind with co-dependent issues as well as my own sick love of anything that I could use to numb out. We got a batch of substance from one of Charlie friends that was actively using again. Charlie placed a little amount for me to use, then he would make his batch ready for injection. Charlie had these huge forearms from working as an arborist for many years in Aroostook County Maine.

He would get all his stuff ready, then proceed to poison himself. I had no clue that the needle was so powerful. Charlie had injected most of the substance, then he broke out in a sweat walked into my bedroom, then "fell out." I went over to him; he opens the window sat on the edge of the bed then slipped like a snail right out of bed. It was so scary for me, I reached for my phone to call 9-1-1 for him but he was already grayish blue. No response at all. I really have to add that if you know someone that is slowing killing themselves with drugs, and by this, I mean if they are actively using any substance, they are just sick and need help and support.

Today I know the difference when someone is serious and when someone isn't about their recovery. Although there are the ones that hide the drugs well.

It's a difficult cycle to break free from. There are days when I think back to remind myself how my addiction got the best of me.

It caused me to have some "drug dreams" for a couple weeks. I didn't realize that how this building would trigger my thoughts. Really since I stopped using drugs, I had stopped having drug dreams altogether. I had detoxed myself from the heroin back in Knox County jail in 2016. That jail felt more like a rehab than a jail. The guards were much more polite than other jails where I had been. When I detoxed from drugs, the time when I was literally poisoning myself with any substance. It took about ten days to physically start feeling better.

Honestly, it wasn't as hard as just changing the thought process of the mind. My body didn't go into extreme shakes. It was harder for me to detox from alcohol than heroin. My body had more of a difficult time detoxing from alcohol, only because I poisoned my body pretty much from vodka for weeks before I decided to stop. Detoxing from anything can be challenging no matter the substance. I think that the only reason I detoxed so easily from heroin is because I didn't use as much because I couldn't afford it. At the end of my "USING," I was only using enough so that I wouldn't feel. Well wouldn't feel mentally to be exact. My addiction was not contained it was causing me to self-harm in any imaginable way you could think. The addict will do anything to avoid detox, imaging doing this for years. I was lucky enough to escape feeding my heroin use at the nine-month mark. The drug grabs ahold of its "PREY" so quickly that they feed into it easily. Especially vulnerable to those who choose not to treat their disease.

Seeing other people injecting drugs in those hallways was a borderline daily nightmare. Actually, not sure why my higher power placed me there but maybe to see more clearly, to understand a bit more while I was awake, rather than drooling all over myself in a lonely attic apartment.

A few weeks later noticed that jack was back at it. To be truly honest with you. The whole situation made me break down and cry for jack. It broke my heart because I could see he was hurting inside but the only way I could help him was to talk to him about recovery and the process.

I believe that when a person is truly serious about trying to live life without substance is when they decide to follow a program and pretty much force themselves to get to meetings. The surroundings of that building jack hardly had a chance to get back on his feet without relapse followed by cycle. Cycle of drugs.

After the overdose I wanted out of the building. I started looking into home ownership. I didn't want to pay rent then have to be stuck with problems. I wanted to take care of my disease so that I could focus more on my recovery. I wanted to be able to just live in a clean safe and quite place. I wanted and craved peace in my life.

This is when I started my research on the homeownership. I had made the step to fix my credit. This meant that I had to face the fact of cleaning up my past debts. I reached out to a place in Orono Maine called four directions. I heard about them from my people at the "WAB" center. I was given a credit councilor to work with me to help fix my credit score. My score was in the high four hundreds at the time, it was bad. I had written a few bad checks a few years back during my active addiction, just to feed my insanity. The desperation of one's illness causes them to do the most harm is when the drugs start to wear off. The lengths that I had went to feed my disease was writing some bad checks which were now haunting me. It's like what was I thinking, I wasn't. I was numb to everything and anything I was pretty much a damaging zombie when I was high on drugs.

When I first sat down to talk about my debts, I was a bit defensive, I was a bit in denial, I was a bit shocked too. I didn't even realize that I took out a credit card with high interest rates just to take them money out so I could get high. I couldn't even pay back the credit card, I had no idea why I decided to get the card to waste away.

I had to clean the mess I created during my drug days. My credit councilor advised me that I needed to pay the banks back for the few bad checks that I had wrote. I had to call to reach out with a payment plan. When a person is first getting sober everything is so hard to do. It's like being reborn or just waking up from coma; it's like having to relearn everything. I was waking up to credit card debt, I knew I had to start cleaning up the mess I had created. Although I wasn't making a lot of money, I decided to do the next right thing by paying the banks back first. I felt angry at first that I had to give my extra spending money away.

Really though it was my own mess to clean, nobody's fault but my own. I had to look at the mess and clean it, so I could move forward.

Getting myself back into financial independence is where I was trying to get myself again. I wasn't happy about having to pay the monthly payments, it's what I needed to get done in order to heal myself. Leaving debts isn't good for anyone. I believe that it's the reason why I was careful in what I was doing when it came to applying for anything. When I was in my unhealthy relationship for years I didn't dare to leave for work because I was afraid to leave my son with his father because of his temper. Back then I was a dependent on him for paying the rent and I was getting assistance from the government.

When I had just had my son, I was interested in going back to school or even just getting a part time job at a store or anyplace that would get me out of the house. My ex would tell me on a weekly basis, 'Melody who's going to take care of the baby while you're gone to work? Back then I didn't understand the power and control wheel of abusive relationships. I just went with the flow to live in peace. I would just say to him "yeah good point." Really, I was dying inside, I wanted to make my own money and be around people. I was kept isolated for a long time in this unhealthy sick relationship. I will get more into that later…

So, after a few weeks passed, I went to see my credit councilor once again. It wasn't as tense as the first appointment. I understood a bit more why I had to make small payments and making regular payments would only benefit me. I noticed just a few months that my credit score started to go up little by little. I was able to make a couple lump payments to my debt collectors. Then my score when up drastically by like fifty points. After the cards where paid, I decided that I would apply for a credit builder card from my bank. My credit councilor advised me to, she became my right-hand advisor. Once I got approved for the credit builder card, I was able to now be able to raise my score monthly. I don't know what I was trying to prove, I knew that having a good credit score would help me get a house loan.

A house, an apartment, a trailer, I was desperate for anything really. Just to be able to escape the apartment house where I was living is what drove me to "escape." Escape from seeing people high or under the influence of some substance. The building was so stressful for me I just wanted to live in peace. I had finished my book and now it was time for me to continue to move forward in my recovery journey.

Home ownership didn't seem realistic to me. I thought that I wouldn't be able to swing it, having to depend on myself 100 percent like that scared the crap out of me. Also, I had so much self-doubt that I could even do anything like this, especially on certain days when my addict mind took over. When I would have my alcoholic thoughts running through my headfirst thing in the morning it was hard. The sick alcoholic mind sends bad thoughts. The disease of self-destruction is what I like to call it now. It's a mind warp at times trying to move forward but the disease of addiction haunts the mind daily with negative self-thoughts and sick thinking. When you hear people saying I'm my own worst critic its what's true about the fellow addict. Therefore, I choose to block out my negative thoughts when I do my daily mediation. Once I knew how to control my thoughts is when the door opens for me. Meditation is what's saved me. I've been able to balance out my days more productively with daily 'prayer walks', is where I talk to my higher power and thank him for another day clean and sober. It's when I wasn't able to control my sick thinking, when I was actively using substance is when I was the most miserable. I realize this today about myself. I was sick once, just to upset myself to start the process of either drinking or getting high. I can say that sometimes I'm able to focus on the things that use to bother me and process them better today. When back a few years ago the "problems" where just extended to cause binge drinking. Well now that I understand my disease a bit more today, I'm able to control what I do and what I say. Anyhow, looking into home ownership was at first scary for me. During my younger days I wanted nothing to hold me down to a certain place. I was a free spirit that just wanted no financial responsibility whatsoever. Thought I knew the best place to protect my recovery was to have a stable and peaceful home. When I was in the process of looking at homes, I was looking at space and neighborhood. I wanted to be close to a grocery store and close to a bus route, just in case my car broke down.

Looking on the outskirts of Bangor is what I originally had in mind. Bangor was a place that I had spent most of my years growing up. I knew the city well; my son wasn't too far away either. My son Anthony was in oldtown at the time living with his father. That was only a twenty-minute car ride at the most, not far at all. Bangor \ Brewer has a great bus system that runs almost daily except for Sundays. The fare is cheap, and the bus drivers are very helpful when needing to find a place. I love taking city buses for some strange reason. I thought if I decided on a house that I would find a spot that I could either walk to work and walk to get my groceries if need be. Also, I wanted to have Anthony to be able to just hop on the bus if he wanted to visit.

One morning on my day off from working at my regular job, yes, I'm an author but I still work because it helps to keep me busy, which is extremely good for a recovering addict. Never get bored, that's when trouble finds you. I knew I had to find a realtor in my area in order to look at some houses. Just so happens Charlie had one of his guitars\ band mates Duane was a realtor. They had known each other even before I knew Charlie. The two of them would work on houses together as well as "jam out" to their guitars. Once when I missed Charlie, the time we were apart I would watch his old videos on his social media pages just to listen to him sing, just to hear his voice. I noticed a few videos when they happen to do a mini concert for Duane's daughter that owns one of my favorite spots in Maine. A campground near Ellsworth called timberland. I knew I wanted to personally meet him; he was artist like myself.

I remember Charlie talking to me about him on a few occasions, I never had the chance to meet him. So, one day out of the blue on a Saturday Charlie says to me, "Melody we are invited to go "jam out" to some music at Duane's. Also, he's a realtor that can help you get a house, he's also my friend"

I said to Charlie, 'ok but I'm not going to sing', he looked at me and spoke. 'Babe you're the writer I'm the singer," we both laughed. The day we went over to Duane's house to "rock out" they had some guest over that were drinking as well. It didn't bother me thought, I knew I would pretty much ruin the party if I drank. I was strong enough in my recovery that I could comfortable just sit and listen to them play and sing. After a couple hours, I felt comfortable and I had enjoyed myself, sober. It's okay to have a little bit of natural fun occasionally.

After that day I knew I found the right realtor, some one that knew the kind of space that we needed in a home. Since we had no children together, we needed only one spare bedroom for Anthony when he visited us on the weekends. I started to look at the websites of houses in the area of Bangor\ brewer I knew that I needed to stay close to my work and to my recovery community. I wanted a place where I could have a small office and a work-out area. Also, a spot for Charlie's guitars and music equipment. A house that could possibly be a forever home to us. I started searching for a house during the winter months of COVID. I came across a few houses in the a few good neighborhoods, houses with a big back yard for family gatherings. I knew that once I got situated that I would start my puppy search. I did want another child but was afraid that my body was too damaged and old to carry. It was a heartache for me for some months knowing I couldn't have another child. My age was a factor with this issue. So, what would ease my heart, a puppy.

We looked at a few houses, but nothing ever matched up. It was out to far from town, a bit run down that would need repair work. So, one day I was looking on the website and came across a beautiful ranch style home close to everything. I emailed the location and numbers to Duane, then he wrote back that we could go look at it that very same day. The house was perfect all except for the kitchen. The day we went to look at the property is when I noticed that it was in the perfect location. The city bus drove right by the street. Also, a nice mini mall was only walking distance from this house. This is when I knew if the house is nice, then we have a winner. Once inside I notice the kitchen was completely old-fashioned, like back fifty years.

I ignored the kitchen and walked around to the living room. It was very comfortable. The bathroom was nice and had been recently remodeled, but the previous owners kept the old tile floors. I walked toward a door that was a small room with a closet and window, alongside another room which had another room. This was the master bedroom connected to a beautiful sunroom area. The sunroom was a beautiful area. It had these beautiful pine wood walls and brand-new windows just recently installed. The room overlooked a beautifully landscaped yard filled with blossoms.

I could see myself doing my daily meditations in this beautiful sunroom. I also envisioned my puppy running in the yard outside. Also, this house had an extra bedroom for my son or a family guest like my parents. That's when I fell in love with the house. I wanted it and I wanted it right away. Anything to escape the nightmare apartment building where I was at would be ideal. But honestly, I never thought I could purchase a house. The only problem that I could see was the kitchen cabinets. The three of us chatted for a moment to figure in some numbers. I looked over to Charlie then said, "I love everything except those darn cabinets." Charlie and Duane looked at each other, then Charlie said, "Honey, I'm a carpenter, I can easily fix that problem." I didn't know that about Duane either. The two of them use to work together flipping\ remodeling houses. It was meant to be then, I looked over to Charlie then said Okay then let's figure this out and place an offer.

I had saved some money for the down payment and moving cost which I knew by the class that I took a few months earlier called "first time home-owner." So, if you're reading this book and you are interested in buying your first home. I do have to suggest, take a first homebuyer's class. The class will teach you everything that you will need to know before and after.

I knew the whole process would take months to complete, so I kept it hush hush. I told nobody except my sister back home in Eskasoni Trudy. The days after I thought about the house and what it would be like to live in a house again. I spent most of my adult years in Maine living in apartment building or renting rooms. I knew though for me to complete my mission to home own-ership was to continue my recovery journey. I couldn't allow myself to get too excited about anything because I could easily get rejected, that could lead to relapse. Honestly anything negative could lead a person to try to escape rejec-tion by "numbing out" on life. I stayed patience and calm during the whole process, I didn't want to fail and fall on my face like I had many times before. What was different this time though was that I had a program that I could rely on daily to keep on track. I noticed that there were more drugs coming into the apartment building and more and more homeless people sleeping in the hallways. It was a very challenging time for me especially during COVID. I cleaned the hallways for the landlord because of COVID and because nobody was doing it. I got along well with landlord. I had built a good friendship with him during the couple years that I stayed at that building. To be completely honest "Andy" the landlord help get me off the streets, so I was like, kind of thankful to him. He mentioned to me the stress that he had about the building that he was trying to sell. I told him one day, "And Andy, I'm actively looking for a home now, but I will make sure to leave this apartment clean for you." He smiled over at me and said, "Well, I've finally had enough of this place, and I can't do it no longer either, kiddo. I'm selling the building. Andy called me "kiddo" for some reason and I didn't mind it.

One morning when I was right in the middle of working, I received a called from Charlie. He had also left me a text message. Once I was able to call him back, Charlie said to me, "They said yes to our offer, Mel. We could get that house." I was so excited I told some of my coworkers. They all knew that I was trying to find a forever home. I had been at this job for a couple years; my coworkers treated me kindly and supported me and my first book. I couldn't wait to get done work that day.

I kind of rushed home, I was so excited jamming out to music and singing in my car on my back home that day. When I got home, Charlie was making us dinner. He had already set the table up and had some chocolates for me. It was nice to have a man that wanted to have a stable home and life again. After dinner we talked mostly about our "what ifs." What if we could move in a couple months? Trust me there was many days when I had packed up my bags and was ready to bail on both Charlie and the building. But I'm a very loyal person that doesn't give up on a person, no matter their past. I had a game plan to start packing up the apartment once we had thirty days to go. The whole home buying process does take some time. It could take months if you don't know exactly what you're doing, so be careful with this.

Once the buyers took our offer and everything fell into place for purchase is when it became easier to live there. Just knowing that I could live at a place without having to worry about who I would have to "bump" into in the hallways. All I wanted was a place to feel mentally and physically safe again.

When a person is just getting clean and sober from substance, it's crucial that they surround themselves with a non-triggering environment. I guess for me I felt strong or some type of invincible to everything around me. Being numbed out from prison and my recent incarceration was enough to set me straight into a floating bubble. I had never been so blocked out from the world before, during my incarceration I found myself in a cell with another inmate for twenty-three hours of the day was enough to set anyone straight into holy-ness.

When I was released from prison, I found myself homeless and without any emotional support. If I had listened to my caseworker Jen in prison, then I would have a much better chance at success. My disease of addiction was calling me even before I was set free that day back in July 2018. Knowing that I could just spend a few days free from watching eyes was when my disease decided to "attack." That's pretty much what happened to me when I decided to go back out and use substance.

I couldn't wait to leave this building where I had been living. There were days that I wasn't sure if could continue on my recovery path. The days when I found myself in my car contemplating my destruction was the scariest times. This happened to me a few times in this building. One of the times is when Charlie had decided to inject Ritalin in to his PICC line, and I had to witness his fast-moving jaw moving side to side instead of the regular movement. Yeah, it sounds scary, because it is scary. When a person that you care about doesn't have the proper self-control with a medication is a living nightmare, feels a bit like babysitting an adult. For my first couple years I had a few occasions that I could had just snuck a six pack of beer or a few pills into my apartment, but I didn't want to. I wanted the clean and sober life. I wanted what the people in the "halls" had. A newfound freedom from self-sabotage to be exact.

The voices I could hear saying, "go out and use just one last time" I kept under control by attending as much self-help meetings and being accountable and honest in all my affairs. I wasn't going to allow anyone, or anything get in my way, even this apartment building. I knew that I could lose everything that I had been working so hard for.

My first year of sobriety when I was waiting for the bus to visit my son in oldtown. I was waiting for the bus inside of the bus station. I was just standing their people watching. I noticed these two young men dressed sharp, walking around towards me. The bus station was crowded, it was midafternoon on a

Saturday. They walked into the bus depot station where everyone was waiting for their buses to arrive. I stood there looked at them for a moment. Then I could notice one of them walking towards me. I had enough street smart to notice when someone wants my attention. I glanced over to the one that was standing closest to me.

He smiled to me, then said, "Hey, beautiful, how are you doing today?" I looked at him and I replied as politely as I could. "I'm doing well today, how about you." He smiled at then gestured his hand to me. I looked at him sideways, with a curious look. I didn't know if he was trying to hit on me or just being extra polite. He went to hand me something in his hand and I took it. Once I looked down to and opened my palm, I noticed a white substance in a small plastic baggie. He said to me, "If you like it, then here is my number. Call me anytime. I have plenty." The flashbacks of a couple years before came back to me. The times when I was buying drugs from random dealers. I placed the white substance into my pocket and told him "thank you, I will." I'm not sure why I placed the substance in my possession. In that moment alone if I were to get caught with this substance, I could get another jail sentence. As a felon, I was in trouble just having this unknown substance on me.

Being so new in my recovery, I fantasized about what this drug was. Was it crack? Was it H? then the insanity took over for a moment. I thought about not visiting my son that day and just going straight home to experiment with it. I stood there in that bus stop for a moment, then I walked outside. Thought about it some more. Then my recovery mind took over once more. I could hear an inner voice telling me to trash this garbage in my pocket. I walked into the public bathroom; then I reached over in my pocket to take a closer look at his white substance. Sure, enough it was crack cocaine, a random stranger just handed me a bag which was probably worth fifty dollars. I could have easily got high for the whole day on it. Then I heard the inner voice once more *"trash that trash, Mel."* I placed the small baggie into the trash can, then I thought, *Well, what if someone gets a hold of it? Then dies.*

I reached over and picked the trash in the bathroom. Some lady walked in as I was picking through this garbage bag. She just gave me a strange look. I felt embarrassed that someone had caught me, I didn't care at that moment thought. Once I seen the small round baggie full of dope, I reached in grabbed the bag. I walked over to where the public toilets were. I opened the package; then I dropped the substance into the toilet and flushed it. What I had just done was almost a gateway to a relapse, but I had remembered and actually reminded myself of how the nightmare life could be in my life once again. I could have easily ruined my recovery time and ruined any good in my life. I wanted to remain on the path, and I wanted to have a good life without substance interference.

After that minor incident at the bus stop. I couldn't help but share the story with a few people. Talking about what I like to call close encounters helps to releases the demon that waits. The demon that waits doing sit-ups is the relapse monster. The inner demon that waits for the exact moment to strike an addict that is vulnerable. The inner demon that haunts our daily lives and wants and waits to take our soul.

After a few weeks passed by the realtor asked me if I had started packing yet. I told him that I had just started to become comfortable with the fact that I was going to become a homeowner. That's when it sank in… I was going to have a nice peaceful place to continue my recovery work. A place where I could start fresh. I was so excited, but I wasn't completely convinced that the work was over. I knew that I might have a few more things to clean up first. After all I was already used to cleaning my side of the street once again with old "things" popping up.

The loan company officer asked me if I was a us citizen. I knew that I wasn't and that I was only able to live and work in the us because I was under a treaty law called the jay treaty. It was signed back in 1794 is an agreement by the United States and Great Britain to allow Canadian born native Americans to travel freely across the United States / Canadian border. I didn't realize the rules as clear as I thought. The papers that the loan company wanted to be completed in order to process the loan were proof that I was legally allowed to live in the United States.

I first had to contact my tribe back in Canada and get an updated native American status card. The card that's as good as a green card when I have crossed the border. While dealing with my tribe for my papers I noticed that

I needed proof of my citizenship and that card would not qualify me to citizenship but just allow me everything else. My emotional roller coaster stared right back up again, I felt as though my dream of home ownership was in jeopardy. I felt as though I wouldn't be able to finish what I had started, and I felt slightly defeated.

My legal citizenship would have to be resolved for me to continue my path to home ownership. I faced it as a challenged that I could place my time on. I contacted my local immigration office in Bangor, the informed me that if I was trying to get citizenship that I would have to drive down to Portland office. I knew that dealing with the state of Maine that I would need some important documents if I wanted to be taken seriously. I tried calling them at first, just to make sure that I didn't waste my time driving down there. I hit a brick wall basically, I couldn't get a real person on the phone. A week had gone by with no call for appointment.

I didn't have the time to just sit back and wait weeks for a call back, luckily for me I was working with an excellent loan officer Luanne. She was one of Charlie's childhood friends, she was very patience during the wait time. I do believe that once she told us that the underwriter was willing to wait a couple more weeks for this loan to get officially approved my inner drive took over once more.

Knowing that I only had a couple weeks to finish this whole process I hit like a blank brick wall. I sat on my bed thinking to myself," how am I going to get the immigration offices attention." I knew I needed help, a person that I could connect me to the main office in Portland without wasting any more valuable time. I called a local representative office in my area of Bangor, along with leaving an email. I was contacted by this office in just a day. I couldn't believe the response I got back; I was able to talk with the representee office people. I told them that I was native American Micmac from Canada trying to buy a house in Maine and that my Indian status card would not be excepted by the loan company, and I needed citizenship as soon as possible. That I only had a deadline of ten days to complete the forms needed. Once the representee knew I had this short period, he gave me his word that he would return my call the following day. Only because he would have to investigate the jay treaty law a bit more.

It's been a whole eye-opening experience for me during my years in Maine, that I'm unable to have my basic native rights in the United States. Once I cross the United States \ Canadian border into Canada my native rights are intact. But as a Canadian native American, I have absolutely none of the privileges that some of my relatives have the comfort of, like healthcare, housing, assistance from government. I'm like the naked Micmac warrior in Maine, naked because I have the same rights as everyone else that's non-native. I've adored the fact that I'm a human and to accept everyone the as an equal person as well, to love all people no matter the difference.

I've learned over the years that I choose to live away from my tribe to better myself and not rely on any form of government assistance only during desperate days. I have even applied for membership to a Micmac tribe in Maine and I was recently rejected by them because I had no relatives there. That was a bit heart breaking for me. I was able to prove my Micmac bloodline and I completed all the necessary paperwork that they wanted just to be rejected by my own people. Trust me when I tell you how painful of a process that was, to be told that I couldn't be adopted by a tribe in Maine was borderline triggering experience. I'm a warrior and I believe in moving forward, I prayed about it and I'm okay today.

The next day my phone rings, nobody usually calls me. I answered the phone, "Hello," then a reply "Hello, Melody, my name is Bradley and I work for the representative office here in Bangor." My heart was pounding, I said to him really? He replied, "Yes, I can understand the situation you are in with this citizenship problem, and we can help you." My anxiety went down a few notches after that. Just knowing that I might be able to find a solution to my problem After all, as a person who is in recovery, it's moments like this that would ultimately cause relapse in our life, especially any form of rejection could create the ultimate excuse to use any substance to numb our feelings. I've done and resorted to this behavior many times over the years.

I was so excited when Bradley told me that I would have the immigration offices in Portland direct phone line, I felt honored. Seriously the response, I couldn't believe how quickly I was helped by this local office. I felt so special that I wouldn't be given a run around, it made me feel special. My emailed to this person in Portland were answered as quickly as io sent them. I called to schedule an appointment, the person that answered the phone was already expecting my call. The moment I called the people at the immigration office were so polite to me on the phone. I was able to get an appointment within a few days. I was able to take a couple days off from work to sort this issue up with the underwriter.

I took the drive down to Portland with my son Anthony. We stayed at the hotel right next to the Portland mall so that we could do some shopping as well. When I was actively using, I didn't care much about sightseeing or taking any mini vacations especially with anyone. We walked around that mall that day for about six hours, just checking out the different stores they had. The food court was nice too.

When Monday morning came, I woke up early at the hotel, went and got some breakfast and coffee then exercised at the gym for a bit just to ease any other anxiety I was having. The gym is so helpful when I need a break from life's struggles. Healthy way to unwind any uncomfortable thoughts that I was having at the time. All I was thinking of was if I would be able to complete my forms correctly. My obsessive thoughts sometimes overwhelming me, it makes it difficult for me to focus.

That morning I drove right to the immigration office. When I walked into the building. I noticed that they had a security guard. The guard greeted me with a smile, then asked if I had an appointment. I looks over at him then said, "Yes, I do." He replied back, "Great." He asked me to sit in a certain spot in the waiting area. I wasn't sure why, but I didn't care. All I knew was that I needed to get this citizenship paperwork figured out so that I could continue moving forward to home ownership. Then my name was called, I looked over to where I was supposed to be. The lady asked me if I had all the necessary paperwork for the application. I wasn't sure at the time, but I thought that I would have to pay an application fee for citizenship. Then after a few moments of polite conversation the lady asked me to take a photo for the card. If I hadn't called the local representative in my area for guidance, I do believe that I wouldn't have been so lucky to get the appointment so quickly. I was handed a temporary citizenship card. To me that was a moment to be proud of, I felt as though I was finally establish.

That afternoon, I took my son for lunch before driving back to Bangor. I talked to Anthony about how lucky we are to be native Americans. That we need to not ever be ashamed of our bloodline.

The following day, I rushed over to my realtor's office, he was able to send the last forms to the underwriter. I wasn't sure if the card would be accepted but all I did know was that I was trying my very best not to give up. I couldn't stand being in that triggering apartment building no longer. After that the realtor told me now, we just wait. I asked about how long this process could take. He mentioned to me that the whole house buying business requires time and patients. Before leaving the office, he said, "Melody, you have done so much to improve your life and lifestyle that this is something you deserve."

Then just like that I felt secure in waiting a few more weeks. It was weird because I was so excited about the house, that I drove by the house every few days. I don't know why I did this, maybe to remind myself that anything is possible once you put your mind to it. I was homeless with nothing but a backpack just a couple years earlier.

Honestly, when I was released from prison for furnishing substance back in 2018. I walked around Bangor for days, I had nothing and no place to go. During those few weeks I would hitchhike down east to spend a few nights on a friend's couch. Those were the days when I thought about why I even existed. That summer I spent a few days at the downtown under the overpass at interstate 395 bridge, where all the other homeless people were. I didn't care exactly who I was with during those few weeks. I was so lost with no shelter. I had been homeless before, so I fit in with them. The strangest part about that time was that I deep down knew I had to make some major life changes or else I would be a chronic homeless forever. That is something that I didn't want, I wanted to be happiness and stability. I had no clue as to what I needed to do.

After a few days the underwriter to let me know that everything had just finished, and all the paperwork was completed and both Charlie and I were approved for the house loan. Charlie was my best friend and partner and I just wanted us both to start our lives fresh. Free from the stressors of that apartment building. We couldn't wait to leave. Then once all the paperwork was finalized, Charlie looked over at me and said, "Honey, we did it, we can start packing now." I was so relieved and felt the same feelings I had when I was set free from department of corrections. Charlie and I embraced, we both had tears of joy. The rewards of changing our lifestyles to be free from substance is what made it possible for this dream to come true. We would be homeowners with a private yard, private mailbox and private everything. The feeling was amazing. Just knowing that I could live in a beautiful neighborhood without any random stranger knocking at the door asking if I wanted to buy something.

This new freedom was overwhelming at first, I do believe that it didn't set in my mind yet. The comfort of just having a quite peaceful home would be so instrumental in aiding my recovery process.

I was having to place my trust with a higher power, I knew that this wouldn't be possible without some form of guidance from the great one.

I had just finished my book to submit and finalize all the editing and cover photo. I had no clue of the publishing process but all I did know is that I wanted to tell everyone what happen to me. I wanted to share with the world that what happen in April of 2017 was an accidental overdose cause by addicts that would not stop the insanity that comes with being an addict and alcoholic. It's something that I don't just move passed, especially knowing that it was someone that I cared for. Georgie is what Charlie called her, his youngest sister. The first time I had ever met G, was in Rockport Maine. I knew her only by social media sites along with phone calls they had. It seemed that they had a close bond, and I had no clue that they shared many secrets with each other. I didn't really know Charlie's family they were a bit isolated from him. I thought that was a sad family dynamic at first, only because I was in regular contact with my family.

I was so excited that day when I could finally meet one of Charlie's family members. I was living in Bangor at the time on grove street in the attic apartment back in 2017. I was doing massive amount of living on the edge with nothing to do except only work a few hours a week, then the rest of the time I drowned myself in self-pity so that I could have an excuse to inject myself with heroin and other substance. I call those days, my nine-month bender of self-abuse. At the time of those days, I was experiencing the love of the needle, that was an addiction to me.

Charlie and I had just finished a weekend of partying on heroin and cocaine. We had run out of money and run out of drugs. We had just started having withdrawal symptoms. Headache, vomiting, massive diarrhea, along with the shakes it's something I don't miss today. Charlie received a phone call from "G" they talked for about a half hour. I could hear Charlie telling her about our crazy weekend of self-destruction. Then Charlie said to me, "Hey, would you like to meet my sister G?" I looked over at him like a mad wife. "I'm not feeling well today. You already know this." He looked at me with the face he gave me when we would be "getting something." He said to me, "She has something that will help us feel better today." I didn't know much about her, only by what he had told me.

I said to him lets go then, any excuse for a road trip for me was well worth it. I was especially excited to be able to talk with someone that was his family. We drove the coastal route from Bangor to Belfast, then Camden then Rockport. If you have driven down coastal Maine before it's a very scenic drive. It took us about 90 minutes to get there. When we drove up to the little house on the side street. I noticed that this house had a huge yard with a doghouse and a few old cars parked. When driving in, I seen Georgie open the front door then waved to us. When she did that, her dog, Ruby, a golden-colored lab, came outside to meet us. I asked Charlie, "Is her dog friendly?" He replied, "Melody, she's friendly." I was still traumatized by the "REZ" dogs that would chase me back home.

Charlie had lived with her for a few months back a couple years earlier so ruby knew Charlie. We walked towards the door; the door opened once again. She said to us, "I'm so glad you two mad it down here to visit me. She greeted the both of us with a huge hug. Then invited us into her home. The house was one of those small cozy cottage looking homes that you would see in movies. She looked at me head-to-toe, then said to me, "Melody, it's so good to finally meet you." I remember so clearly the look she gave me with the most beautiful smile I hadn't seen in years. Her eyes where a deep ocean blue on a sunny day. She was a female version of Charlie, and I couldn't believe the similarities they shared.

She looked at me again and gave me this devilish smile, then said, "I can't believe you're so beautiful, are you Native American. The line I usually received when just first meeting someone. Then I proudly said to her, "Yes, I am Micmac from Eskasoni." We both laughed and asked each other questions for a few moments. It was almost like we already knew each other. I felt this closeness to her in just a few minutes. I guess that's what people sometimes call "instant connection."

Then after we conversed, after about forty-five minutes. She looked over at Charlie, then said, "Let me go and get my Ritalin for us to take." She asked Charlie to stop and get fresh needles at the store on our way over. Charlie took out the "supplies" to use for injection, which usually consisted of a spoon, a band, water, then the substance. I was sitting at her kitchen table and she handed me ten Ritalin and a bit of heroin then said, "This should make you feel a better." We all took some to inject ourselves. After we finished our sick behavior, I noticed a few guitars in the living room. I looked over at Georgie, then said to her with a big smile on my face, "Do you play guitar as well?" She had this, like, vibe to her that was almost rockstar. She had given me that look of what do you think? Then replied, "Yes, I can play and sing too." She grabbed her guitar, a blue Epiphone that had these musical notes on it.

She asked me, "What would you like for me to sing for you today?" I said to her, "Anything you want." Once she started to sing, I couldn't believe the unbelievable talent that came out. She sang some '80s country songs for us. Then Charlie, of course, took over and sang as well. We jammed out to the music, then continued to party that afternoon away. We took a drive to Walmart, then picked up some pizza for dinner. After dinner Georgie asked if I wanted to stay for the night. That she was lonely and fighting depression. I could tell that she enjoyed visiting with me, it was a pleasure for me as well. Getting to know her I found it interesting the similarities that her and Charlie shared. Being a native American our culture teaches us to stay connected with family. Family is the most sacred part of being a native, it's the most important tradition to share with our children, staying connected with loved ones, no matter the situation.

Georgie, looked over at me with her deep blue eyes, then said, "Melody, it was so nice to finally meet you. I hope to see more of you from now on." she sat next to me, then we talked for another thirty minutes of so. Talking about life and our war stories mostly.

She mentioned to me how close she was to her parents, that they had passed away and how she longed for them. A part of me wanted to just stay there in Rockport with her, I liked the way she talked.

I had to work the next morning so we couldn't stay even if we wanted to.

After that day, we all would get together to use and abuse substances frequently. Even when Charlie got very sick that winter with a condition called endocarditis, we still would all party together. A few weeks after Charlie got out of the hospital in Boston. We drove down to Rockport to pick her up so that we could visit and party. We arrived to get her in early afternoon, she had with her a light overnight bag. I didn't care that she would spend a few days with us, I just thought that we would visit as well.

Once we arrived back to Bangor Georgie asked us if we could get some heroin for the weekend, she wanted enough to last a couple days for the three of us. I thought it was a bad idea at first. All I could think of was Charlie taking too much again. That for me was very stressful, I didn't want him to die again. After all he had just came back from Boston a few weeks earlier from an infection in his heart caused by injecting himself with needles. But when a person is in active addiction, thinking things out is hardly an option. Pure insanity is what I'd like to call it. Irresponsible behavior caused by poor decision making, is ultimately the perfect storm of self-destructive behavior. It's like rational thinking doesn't occur when a person is high on substance. The only thing that's going through an addict's head is obsessing over this drug.

After a few hours back in Bangor we finally were able to get ahold of one of the couples that regularly provided our drugs. When she decided to buy a couple grams of what we thought was heroin, I knew that something bad could come of this. I had experienced these nervous feelings I was having, almost every time when buying a large amount 0f drugs. I just shut my mouth; I didn't want to start any unnecessary arguments that weekend. She was so excited to just spent time with us, not only to party but visit as well. When we got back to the apartment that night. None of us overindulged; it was like we only did enough to get physically comfortable. This is the insanity of these nasty drugs, you want it just to get back to feeling a bit normal, pure insanity.

We ended up going shopping that night for groceries and a few other things. I remember this shopping trip so vividly, well because the each had one of those special motorized carts in the store. I was walking alongside the two of them. At one point they did race each other down the aisle, laughing so hard that it drew other customers attention.

I thought the whole thing was a bit strange. Georgie had picked up some hair dye so that we could color our hair that night. It was funny because she picked my color and I picked hers. After months of getting to know each other, I cared deeply for her, I was adopting her into my life. We colored each other's hair that night. We all stayed up until sunrise just getting high and talking about life. We all just ended up making breakfast and having coffee.

We gathered in the living room area, to start preparing to feed our nasty habit. After I looked at what Charlie had in his spoon, I got angry, then said, "He can't have that much, he will die" they both looked over at me then removed some. After he sat down near the bed, he injected himself, then started to "nod out." I didn't think much of it at the time because I was so used to seeing him high, that it didn't faze me. After a few minutes of feeling the effects. I noticed Charlie was in a laying down position with his eyes shut. I reached over in a panic. "Charlie, are you okay?" He didn't reply. I looked over at Georgie than said, "I think he's overdosed again." We both panicked mostly because we didn't want him to die. I reached over to get my cell phone then called 911. He was just lying there turning that grayish blue color again. While waiting for the emergency units to arrive.

I knew that it could be possible that Charlie could have added more to his spoon when I left the room for just one second. I couldn't believe how fast he dropped out on us.

It was so scary; then I asked her, "Did he add more?" She didn't know what to say. We both yelled at each other in blame, we didn't say pleasant words to each other, it was horrible. We both knew that the police would be coming as well, so we both cleaned up all the evidence as quicky as we could. Even in that moment when my fiancé and her brother was in the other room dying, we thought about our "drugs first," how sick and disturbing is that. That is as sick as it can get when you are in active addiction and don't have the desire to stop.

Then my cell phone starting to ring, I answered it right away. I heard the sirens from the third floor arriving near us. I knew they might have trouble finding which apartment door to enter. The building had four doors in front, so I knew that I would have to run downstairs to meet them. I ran outside I noticed two police cars. I walked to police officer, then said, "Please help us. He's upstairs and unconscious." The police officer looked at me, then said, "Where is he?" I noticed the ambulance arriving and more police. I had them all follow me up to the third floor. This apartment was on the third floor, an attic apartment. Once I got back upstairs, I noticed Georgie was sitting next to Charlie saying "Please don't let my brother die." The police asked me what and when did he take the drugs? I lied and said he went for a walk to meet someone; then when he returned, he collapsed on the bed. How insane that was for me to just blatantly lie about this makes me sick today. I could have easily told on myself, but I wasn't ready. I wasn't ready to give up this crazy lifestyle that I was on. This insane roller coaster ride I was on, a ride worse than the Excalibur.

The police officer gave him a shot of Narcan, then waited a few minutes. Charlie was on the floor already gray. It looked as though it was too late. After a couple minutes passed, there was no response. The police officer looked over to the paramedic, then said, "What now?" The paramedic's response was quick—give him another dose of Narcan.

After that second shot Charlie didn't wake up, but he did start to breathe again. He didn't open his eyes, but he started breathing again. There was a state cop, four police officers, and two paramedics and what looked like an undercover cop. It was so strange all of them just waiting for Charlie to wake up. His breathing sounded unnormal it was more like a loud snore. He did this for about ten minutes. I went in the living room then thought to myself, *What if he doesn't wake up? Then what?* I lose my best friend. I was scared. I walked back in the bedroom, and they had given him another dose, so, yeah, three shots of Narcan. He finally started to open his eyes, once he noticed all the people around him, he said, "Where is she, where my wife?" I looked over at him, then said, "I'm right here, Charlie. I was so scared that you were going to die, you almost didn't wake up." He sat up confused looking. "What happened?" The police told him, "Charlie, this is the third time we have revived you in the past year. When are you going to stop this?"

The paramedics insisted he be admitted to the local hospital so that he could get help that he needed. Then he politely asked everyone to leave the apartment.

Once the room was empty with just the three of us, Charlie asked me, "Where is the rest of the drugs, Mel?" I was the one who had hidden it so the police wouldn't take it, so that I could use it myself. This is how powerful and sick a person thinks when substance is involved. All the addict wants is that "high feeling." Chasing that feeling is what becomes the daily obsession.

Part of the reason why I didn't want to give it back to them is because I wanted to control how much would be taken each time. Seriously, how insane is that? When an already sick person doesn't want to give it up because they don't want the drugs to run out again, only because they want to stretch it out as much as possible. Pure insanity is what most people would call it—chasing a high that cannot be matched usually followed by some sort of accidental overdose or worst...death. When I decided that I would only "manage" the drugs and how much at a time would be taken. I was thinking that if only I gave the drugs back in small amounts so another overdose wouldn't happen. I knew it wasn't mine, but at the time, it was my apartment. Charlie became really agitated toward the both of us.

I sat down to talk with him for a moment; I had no choice really. He had blocked the door so I wouldn't leave. He demanded to know where I had "stashed" the other portion of what was left over. Charlie was all pale-looking with sweat pouring from the side of his face. He looked over at me again then said, "Melody, please tell me where you put the rest of the heroin." I could tell that he was ready to fight or flight if I didn't tell him. I looked over to him then said, "Just look at yourself for a minute, Charlie. You almost just died from taking too much." He shook his head then said, "I know, maybe I should have just died." My heart sank for him. His sister G was in the other room; then he whispered… "Melody, please I'm not feeling good." I looked at him them yelled at him, "Charlie, it's because you had to be Narcan-ed four times before you came back this time." He shook his head and then went to talk with his sister in the living room. This was the time that Charlie scared me, I didn't want him to die. After a few hours and a nap. I had hidden the rest of the drugs in the bathroom on the floor wrapped in a dirty sock in plain sight.

I reached over to open the bag of substance then reached then handed back to Georgie, here is the rest of your "stuff." I didn't want to be there anymore with them, so I took a long walk. I had no place to go

I thought about all the times that Charlie had close call and that I was living with someone that possibility wouldn't change. I honestly thought about my "old life" the life I had with my ex and how I missed the stable life of motherhood. I walked for about three hours that evening, in Bangor. My feet where wet and I was cold, I had to go back to the apartment. Once I went upstairs, I noticed them talking at the kitchen table. They were talking about their childhood and sharing trauma stories. I walked into my room; I closed the bedroom door behind me. I changed out of my wet clothes, then lay on my bed for a few hours. Charlie sat on the edge of the bed then said, "Melody, I'm sorry for fighting with you about the drugs." At the time I just hated him and how I was living my life. I was upset at myself and upset about the way things were going. I really wasn't happy.

I wanted to be normal again and not addicted to the needle and the substance. I wanted out of the insanity of the lifestyle the drugs, but I didn't know how to stop. I didn't have any friends that I could call and have a normal conversation with. I had pushed all my sober and clean people out of my life to make room for "drug friends, drunk friends." I had nobody I had nothing. I had family but hey were back home. I had lied to them for months, my family thought I was still clean and sober and that I hadn't had such a bad relapse. Before this "nine-month drug binge," I had almost three years without substance. The only problem during that time was that I wasn't completely in a "program."

Charlie said, "Do you want a shot of some," looked over then said 'sure, because I don't want to get sick." It's g I was scared of the so-called nightmare withdrawal of this nasty drugs. Scared to be normal or scared to face the reality of this life I had started with Charlie of daily substance use. I looked over to Charlie the only way I will take a shot is if you both don't take too much. I felt as though I was babysitting when we had these "drug parties." After that night of party with Georgie, it was Sunday morning and I was sitting in the kitchen, Georgie walked into the kitchen to talk with me. We both had coffee and made some breakfast. Finally, we were doing something that was normal, making breakfast and talking about life. She called a friend to pick her up that day and she left the rest of the drugs with me.

Today, when I look back at these days and feel so grateful that I don't chase substance anymore. After a few weeks we ended up doing the same old drug chase for weeks. Instead of getting help for us, we just kept doing the same song and dance of the drug shuffle.

Then in April, 2016 Charlie's sister Georgie called me, she said, "Hi, Mel. When are you going to visit me again?" It had been at least a month since Charlie had the close call with death. I told her that I couldn't do much because I didn't have a legal automobile. I had let the insurance and registration expire because I wanted to feed my addiction rather than keep up with my bills.

After I thought about it for a few, she said to me, "Melody, I can give you half of what you get me."

At the time I was so desperate to maintain my daily habit that I was already doing things for money to get high, so this was easy compared to what I had to do. Selling my soul, selling what I could to feed this monster inside of me. The sick things an addict isn't proud to do but too desperately sick to know the difference. I feed the monster once more, I agreed to get some substance for her so that I could use the drugs. Thinking to myself that I was doing a good, but the reality of the situation is that I was feeding the zombie inside of me. Providing someone drugs thinking that I was doing good for someone is as sick as it gets. I had no clue what and why I was doing these things except I was sick addict trying to feed my habit. I met her halfway that day. She sent the money via bank and directly deposited into my bank so I could buy the drugs then meet her halfway was the plan.

It was mid evening and I had Charlie drive, in our illegal auto halfway to Rockport. She was meeting us halfway. It was a quite ride down, we didn't say much to each other. Charlie wasn't too excited about how we planned it all out. He basically was along for the ride. We parked at the spot we all agreed on. We sat there for about fifteen minutes; then we seen headlights from a distance. She had driven herself halfway to meet us. Once the exchange was made, we left and drove back home. She messages me that night telling me how much she loved me and that I was her new "little sister." I had no clue as to what was about to happen.

The next morning, I had to get up early for work. I was only working less than twenty hours a week. I would usually work early first shift do I was up early. Just before leaving I heard Charlie phone ringing. He didn't get up to answer it so I looked over to see who it might be so early. It was a missed call from one of Charlie's relatives, I knew in my hear that it wasn't going to be good news. I woke Charlie up right away, "Hey, Charlie, hey, Charlie, someone from your family called you." He looked up at me then said, "Okay, Mel. Thank you."

Charlie returned the phone call it was one of his siblings, telling him that tragic news about G. She had passed away the night before and that the boyfriend she was living with found her unconscious. After Charlie and I both broke down, knowing that she might have been using alone and that she took too much with nobody there to watch her. But the way it sounded was that the police were going to do a full investigation on where she had got the drugs. A normal person would have walked away from the drugs forever at this point. Charlie was so distraught. I couldn't leave him there alone, so I called into work that day. It was difficult for me to see Charlie so upset; I couldn't imagine the pain that he was going through. I knew her but I didn't have the connection that they shared. So instead of grieving like normal people, we thought about numbing out again. We ended up using all the rest of the drugs that day.

The next day we had a serious conversation about what had just happened. We didn't know what was going to happen next. All I knew was that I had provided someone with a drug, and they overdosed and that's something that I knew would have to live with for the rest of my life. This is something that hurts me today.

I made a choice to leave the substance alone but only for a few days, until I stared to get and feel the effects of the drugs leaving my body. I thought that I would be able to move on and just start making changes. But really, I was only fooling myself, I was isolated from the community at this point. I had no real friends. I didn't even have the support from my family because they didn't know what I was doing. What I was really doing was getting high daily and not allowing anyone to see what I was doing. It was obvious to see, if you really knew me back then. I wore long sleeve shirts to hide my arms. I rarely ate any food; I was pale looking, and I couldn't look anyone in the eye.

Basically, I was a walking zombie, a person that wanted to only get the drink or drug so that I could continue to live in a denial state and zone out. My life was a mess, I had nobody that I could reach out to. I was in a state of mind that was just sick, and I wanted to die at times. I was afraid to ask for help, I was afraid to go to public places, fear of being judged or hated. I had just felt this tremendous load of guilt from what happened to Charlie's sister. When the guilt and shame would come creeping in, this is when my inner monster would come out to haunt me, haunting my thoughts, haunting my soul, haunting even my spirit especially.

After a few weeks of using drugs daily to numb out of any feelings I was having. I was in a depressed state. Charlie was more depressed than I had ever seen him before. I felt horrible inside for how I let my life get so insane.

I was still working but only part time, I wasn't making enough money to pay the bills and Charlie was using all his money for drugs. The rent was way pass due and we just let all of the bills go. We had talked about the possibility of the drug enforcement agency getting ahold of us to press charges on us for the overdose. The chance that we would be sent away became real. I never imagined myself being locked away for a long time. I hadn't even done time before. The only type of isolation from the public that I ever had was rehab. That was back in 2012 when I had to do a court ordered treatment in order to get my son back from the state of Maine.

I was very scared, I had thoughts of running away back to Canada and never returning. I knew that I couldn't leave my son. The son I had not seen for over a year. The pain of not having him in my life daily was the reason I decided to use substance to numb out all my feelings. I had already done nothing to improve my lifestyle. I had destroyed my life in just a year, a year of binge drinking, binge using drugs.

A part of me wanted to be, I hated how I was living. I was tired of being sick all the time. I just didn't know what else to do but to continue the sick cycle of drug dependency.

This one morning I woke up next to Charlie. It was about eight thirty in the morning. I knew we had no food and no drugs to get us going. I decided to call an old friend of mine from down east Maine, a friend that I had known all my life really because he was a friend of the family. Everyone knew him by the nickname made famous by native Micmac from the Maritimes "Cadillac Bob." I had met Bob when I was just a young girl. My mother had been friends with him since they were teenagers. They would work together in the Blueberry Barrens back in the '70s, '80s, and '90s. Bob always treated me like a long-lost daughter. He was a friend of mine since I got re acquainted with him back in the summer of 98.

I would call Bob regularly to check on him and to check in with him. He was friends with some of my relatives and he kept in regular contact with them as well. I knew that I could make a few extra dollars doing some house chores for him. I made the call, the phone rang for a few minutes, then I heard Bob answer, "Hello?" I replied, "Hi, Bob, how are you doing? He replied, "I'm doing well, Melody." He then replied with "How about you?" I said that I was doing fine. I was lying. I was too ashamed to tell him about my recent relapse and my new drug of choice. He replied, "Well, I haven't heard from you in a while. What have you been doing these days?" I told him that I was good, but that I was needing to make some extra money for groceries. Bob said he could help me.

I woke Charlie up with some coffee, then told him that I was going to take a drive down east to clean up for Bob. I asked Charlie if he wanted to come along, but he declined. So, I gathered some spare change that I had around the house to put in the gas tank. I was taking a chance just driving this truck down east from Bangor. The registration was due, the insurance was due, the truck needed an oil change as well. All of this didn't matter to me. I knew that I was about to run out of drugs that's we had been stretching out for days. Only using small amounts at a time, just so we wouldn't have any withdrawal symptoms. Pretty desperate when I look back on it today. I honesty just gave myself a panic attack just thinking back to these nightmarish days.

I had been able to put like eight dollars' worth of gas in, probably just enough to make it down the airline road gas station. As I was driving down there, I had this overwhelming feeling of turning the car back around. I just had this strange feeling that I should just turn back. I pulled the truck over in in Clifton. I didn't know exactly what was bothering me but a part of me didn't want to keep going. I sat there for about twenty minutes. Then I thought about Charlie, so I called him. When he answered his phone. I asked him, "Do you want me to come back home and just forget the job?" He said, "No, Melody, we don't even have any milk or food." We both knew that I was only getting money so that we could spend like maybe twenty dollars on food the rest would go to drugs.

That was the reality of my daily life back then. I like to call this the zombie days of destruction. I ended up driving all the way to Cherry field. I was in the middle of cleaning when Bobs telephone rang. I just kept doing the dishes like I would always do. Bob answered the phone. Then he looked over at me. "Melody, it's for you." I looked at him weird. "What, really?" I looked at the caller ID and it was Charlie's phone. My cell phone didn't usually work down East in certain areas. I didn't know what was up with Charlie. I said, "Hello, everything okay?" He replied, "No, not really." I said, "Well, I will be driving back home soon, so order us some 'medicine.'" Then Charlie replied with a low tone, "I can't do that today, Melody." I wondered why he was saying this to me, then I asked, "Why not, Charlie? What's going on?" He remained silent for a moment then said, "Remember when I told you that the DEA would come question us about my sister's death?" I started to feel panic. "Yes." Then he replied back to me, "Well, Melody, they are here at the apartment with me now and I'm being arrested for trafficking drugs. They want to talk with you as well."

I was in disbelief at first. I first became angry at him. "Why did you answer the door in the first place? Charlie handed the phone to a drug agent; I could hear them talking in the background. I couldn't believe it. The DEA said to me, "Melody, I know exactly where you are right now, so it's best if you could just come back to Bangor and turn yourself in." I said to him, "Turn myself in for what? What did I do?" He said to me, "We know that you and Charlie were the last ones to see G alive." I knew that I had rights, so I told him that I would be turning myself in that afternoon after I took care of a few things, pretty much to get my fix of drugs before I would be brought to jail. When I hung up the phone. My hands where shaking. Bob asked me, "Everything okay, Mel?" I sat down and told him the truth about what I had been doing. He sat there and just listened to me talk for the next hour. I told him that I had to be back in Bangor that afternoon, or I would have a warrant. I asked Bob if I get bail if he could bail me out, poor Bob said he would if it wasn't too much.

Once I knew that I was heading to jail anyways, I decided that I would stop at my dealer's place in Brewer. My dealer at the time was an old coworker of mine. She was on bail conditions and wasn't supposed to be doing anything wrong. She was facing five to eight years for trafficking drugs. She was caught with $25,000 cash and another $10,000 in heroin. She had been on bail for over a year and was living with her mother-in-law in Brewer. Once I got back into town and talked with her, I told her what had happened and that I had to turn myself in that evening, but I wanted to get high first. I bought just a small amount to use before I went home. I sat there and talked with her and visited for a couple hours. Talking about the different scenarios that could come of this.

Then I finally drove back to my apartment, I shut all the lights off and cleaned the apartment up a bit, in case I wasn't going to return right away. Then I called the DEA agents to come get me. They were polite enough to let me take care of few things first, so I kept my end of the bargain as well. I heard loud police knock on the door, you know that type of knock that gets everyone's attention. I yelled to them, "The door is unlocked." Once they came in, they asked me if I had anything on me, I had just thrown everything that we used in the dumpster outside. They handcuffed me, then they read me my rights. I was placed in a regular looking car with tinted windows in the back.

It was an undercover car. When we got on the road the main detective asked if I was interested in becoming an undercover informant. I wanted nothing to do with telling on anyone, so I just kept quiet. I asked about Charlie and where he was. They said they had already booked him in the Knox County jail earlier that day. They also started asking me questions on who was supplying the drugs to us but still I refuse to answer the questions because I knew I had the right to remain silent, so that's what I did.

When I arrived at the jail. I didn't know what to expect. I was still little high from earlier and I had noticed Charlie directly across the booking area from me. I noticed that he was in orange jumpsuit, like a onesie. I just waved to him, and I noticed that he was trying to get my attention again. The guards covered his booking area with a blanket so that we couldn't see each other.

After I was booked, I noticed that there was a small cell with no bathroom in it. It was the holding cell, the place where they asked every question before your in general population. Also, this was the general protocol with new inmates. Searched and observed. I asked the guards when I can get some medication because I've been using drugs steady for months. The guard looked at me then said, "You will see the nurse after dinner." She will check all your vitals and give you something for the discomfort of the withdrawal. I started to feel sick already and it had only been a couple hours in the tiny cold booking room. I just covered my head with the blanket and went to sleep for a few hours.

When I woke to hear my name being called, "Paul, time for meds" that's when I knew that I needed to get up. I sat up then walked near the guard. He escorted me towards to nurse's station. Then once again I passed by Charlie then waved to him. The guard said, "Don't do that please." I replied back to him, "That's my boyfriend." Then he said, "Yes, I already know that, but you two are also codefendants now, so that means no contact." I had never been to jail before, and I certainly didn't know how to respond to much. All I knew was that I needed some medications. I was afraid of what would happen to me if I didn't have any. It had been months of binge using and I hadn't gone more than a day with a substance. It was pure hell really, thinking back on how I lived back then makes me sad for my old self.

After I was done talking with the doctor, I was able to get some medications right away. They gave me a combination of pills that made me feel a bit relaxed and not so anxious. Something I wasn't expecting. They placed me in a larger cell with a toilet and gave me some reading material and writing paper. I started to write down some things, mostly my name and what I was going to do when I would be set free. I was in a bigger room and across from me I could see other inmates.

This is when my detox started, the jail placed me on a liquid diet for the first twenty-four hours. I was uncomfortable, my thoughts were not clear, and I started the process of "repair." I say repair only because this is how I feel about coming off the dope. The poison exits the body slowing but repair starts taking place in the mind and body.

It didn't take me long until I started to feel anxious and overwhelmed about how my life was going at the time. I had been on a nine-month long bender, with only one other worry on my mind. Drugs. It wasn't what I wanted but it was my medicine of numbness for the nine months that I couldn't even remember that life outside of drugs did exist.

Being in this cell alone meant that I was also there with the reality of my life and thoughts. It was my own little detox of bad dreams followed by the reality of my life. I had been avoiding fighting custody with my ex for visitation rights. Therefore, I had not seen or talked to my son in about a year and a half at that point. I didn't bother to follow with the courts. I was just so torn and broken about this major life change that I failed to do the most important thing a parent could do, selfcare.

I failed to be a responsible parent for almost two years, the guilt and shame that followed was a reminder that my life was unmanageable and a mess in every way possible. Now to top it all off, I had these new legal problems that I was facing possibility of years in prison.

I was living a full-on nightmare. This is when I believe that I that I came to a belief that I needed help from a higher power.

In all the years I spent being in a controlling, mentally abusive relationship with an ex. This was something larger than any nightmare scenario I could have created in my own head. In that jail cell I experienced withdrawal not as harsh as I have heard other people describe detox. I had already experience withdrawal from opioids and benzos, this wasn't as bad as what I had experience before. I knew that I could have "meds" and that they were keeping a close eye on me, so I didn't care as much.

After the fourth day I started to feel like myself again. I felt as though I could be myself and leave the jail. I started on regular jail foods. This jail treated me like a human, back in those days I didn't surround myself with people that wanted to recover.

I felt as if I was slowly melting away all the substances from my body. The drugs leaving my system was the answer that I needed back then. The jail finally placed me in a common area of the jail with other inmates. It looked like a collage dorm room, the floors even had carpet with regular wood doors, not mental. The "dorm" had six rooms, four of them with bunk beds, two that were single rooms. I was lucky enough to get a single room. Maybe they knew that I wasn't completely detoxed. I was in this "dorm room" for about three days. The jail had programs like meetings, bible study, gym, school programs. A classroom for the inmates that were interested in completing school or taking their high school equivalency (GED).

On the third day, I was called for court to face my charges. I was sent back to the holding area, where I was booked. There were four other females with me. I had made a friend named Kathleen. She was kind to me, always answered questions that I had about the jail. I guess she had been there a couple times before. The staff even knew her nickname—"Kaz." Kathleen had a good way about her. Her personality could draw everyone in the room's attention with her humor. While getting ready for transport to the courthouse, we all noticed the five inmate males in shackles across the hall from us. Everyone said they were due for court as well.

Then I noticed one of them was Charlie. It was hard not to notice him. He towered over most of the other guys, tall and bulky built. I waited to make eye contact, then he noticed me too. He smiled at me then made some signs that I couldn't really understand. Then, we all were in the same room together. The transport guard gave us a talk, mostly stating, "No funny business while in transport or we could press charges." The transport van was larger than a usual van, enough to have ten passengers.

There were cages in between the seats, so we couldn't hug or anything. I sat right behind Charlie, this is when I asked, "Charlie, how are you doing with the detox?" He tilted his head then said, "I'm doing okay, honey." The van ride was short about five minutes, we were able to talk about what could happen. Charlie talked about our charges. That normally people that face a drug trafficking charge get four or more years at the minimum. This is when I knew that we might not be together again for a while after today. Once we arrived at the courthouse, they placed us all in a waiting area. Everyone was unsure of their faith, the half of us were in there for drug related charges. It was just the first arraignment.

All that I can say when I look back on this time is that I'm happy I'm not in a situation like this today. I didn't know how everything would go in court. I didn't have a clue as to what exactly I was facing for jail time either. All I do know today is that it was a horrible but great learning experience.

Everyone in court had a chance to speak with an attorney.

When it was my turn to speak, the judge looked at me from top to bottom. I looked up at the judge, then when she read the charge of aggravated trafficking. This is when I felt like I was going to throw up, I imagined myself going into convulsions right there on the spot. But that wasn't the case, I answered her as politely as I could. She read, "Miss Paul, do you understand the charges filed against you?" I replied, "Yes, I understand." Then the state had a moment to share the case with her. After he read what they had placed me under arrest for, what they decided to charge me with was aggravated trafficking of drugs.

As I stood there listening to what they had come up with, is when I felt as though my life would never be the same. I didn't intentionally try to hurt anyone; I was not in my right frame of mind. I felt remorseful and shameful when I heard what the district attorney was reading about me.

I looked over at the other inmates, then I shook my head in absolute disgust. I felt sick to my stomach and felt as though my life would never be the same again. I had put myself in this insane drug induced coma for nine months. This was the "thaw out" period. As I stood in front of the judge realizing that this was a hundred percent result of my disease, my disease of addiction.

I had a moment of clarity for the first time in almost a year. I knew that I needed to be locked away for a little bit. To clear myself of substance. I wanted a life free from drugs and the insanity of my disease of addiction. I didn't have a clue as to where I was going in life, I didn't really have a life.

When my lawyer asked me, "Melody, do you want to ask for bail at this time?" This is when my disease took over. I replied, "Yes, bail," so that I could go on one more extreme bender before I had to surrender myself to the state. Honestly that is what I was thinking of, to just numb out for days and days. When it came time for the lawyer to speak on my behalf, he asked for bail. The judge said, "Bail is set to ten thousand." I looked over to the lawyer then said, "I can't afford that. Please ask if it can be reduced." The lawyer then said, "Melody can't come up with that amount. Can the bail be set lower?" This is when the judge said to me, "Melody, I can set the bail to five thousand." Then I said, "That's too high." She then said, "Well, Miss Paul, what exactly where you thinking of?" I said to her, "I could afford a $500 bail with conditions." The lawyer spoke again, saying, "Melody isn't a felon and hasn't been in any major trouble in her life." The judge looked over at me, then said with a serious tone, "If I set bail for five hundred with bail conditions with drug court/substance abuse counselling, can you do this?" I replied, "Yes." I was lying and I wanted out.

That is when I got my chance to get back out and try to take care of myself. Part of me was scared, part of me wanted out of that jail cell, part of me wanted to use substance. The other inmates were not given lowered bail. I think I was given lower bail because I had the part time job, also that I was not a felon.

Once we all returned to the jail, I was told that I could make a phone call to get "bail." I called my friend Cadillac Bob first to tell him that I was in Rockland and that I needed to be bailed out. Bob always knew what to say and what not to say. The phone rang a few times before he picked up. Then I heard him pick up. "Hi, Bob." He said, "Hi, Melody, how are you?" Then I said to him, "Well, I'm in jail and need bail." He then asked me how much? I said to him five hundred, then said, "Please, Bob, I will pay you back. I promise." I could hear that he took a deep breath then said, "Okay, but I can't do much until Monday." I was so excited that I would be able to be free.

I waited out the five days, the rest time was much needed. That morning I was given another free phone call, so I called Bob. Just to see if he was planning to bail me out and give me a ride back home to Bangor.

I had nobody that I could really depend on in the states. Bob was the only person that always had my back in all my good times and bad, he treated me like a long-lost daughter at times. When the phone rang, Bob picked up quickly this time. He said to me, "Hi, dear. I'll be on my way shortly." Then I said to him, "Thank you so much, Bob, I love you." Then he said, "I love you too, kiddo, my pain-in-the-butt daughter." Then we both laughed. Bob arrived at around five; then by the time I was officially "set free" was about six.

On the drive back, we talked about what could happen and what I had been doing. He was understanding as usually and pretty much listened to me talk the whole way back to Bangor. The next day I had to do my first check-in with the courts. The court placed me a strict pre- release bail, so I had to call them daily also I had to check in weekly at the jail. Once I got back to my apartment, I thought about drinking again. I knew that I couldn't because I would be violating my bail and could be sent back to jail, something I wasn't interested in doing.

The next morning, I wasn't sure what I would be doing to "fix" my problems. Honestly if I knew back then what would have helped me the most is a twelve-step meeting. I was clueless and I really didn't care to save myself at the time. All I thought about and continued to obsess about was getting as "wasted" as much as I could. Those first few weeks where I had to check in with the prerelease caseworker was nothing but a show for me. I really had no interest in changing my life for the better. I wanted to be set free so that I could continue to cause damage and destruction in my life, unmanageable to the max.

A few days after my release from jail, I went to where I was working at the time. Just to be told that due to my charges that I had to be temporarily "laid off" from my job of five years, this hurt me a bit. At the time I was only working part time maybe twenty hours, but it was a job. After being told that I couldn't work, I thought about the "binge" once again. As I walked home that day, all I wanted to do was either get high or drunk. I didn't have the mind set to change my path. I didn't allow myself enough time to heal from the destruction of substance to even think clearly.

As sad of a situation that I created for myself, I hadn't felt so beat in my life. I knew that there was a slight chance that I could face prison time if I didn't follow the rules of this bail conditions. The bail conditions kept me away from substance for maybe a week or two. Once I figured out how to manipulate the court system. This is when I started my major last bender.

Honestly, as I sit here in my home office so early on a Saturday morning. I'm thinking back to all the crazy times and it's causing me slight anxiety, I won't lie. It's necessary to share this because it's my breaking point.

I had gone about a week and a half of being clean without any substance. I was in a "crave mode" I was trying to look for any excuse to either get high or drink so that I could just "numb out." After I had just finished talking to the caseworker to give her an update as to what I was planning to do with my life. I had no plans to work on my life. I didn't have enough power to control myself. I was an addict/ alcoholic left alone in an attic apartment. I was alone, scared, depressed to the max.

I didn't have the tools or will power to face my life back then. I just wanted to throw the towel in every chance I got, to continue my self-sabotage. At that point I was merely looking for any excuse to start my bender of destruction. I had enough money to get a few malt beverages, so I planned it out. I planned it out so that I would start my drinking after my nightly check-in with pre-release caseworker. I planned this like a normal person planned a date. This is how quickly my drinking obsession started, I protected my secret drinking like it was my mistress. Pure insanity took over, as soon as I hung up the phone with the worker. I walked to the corner store to get myself a couple malt beverages.

I walked back to my apartment as though I only had food in my bag. It's weird but I would always buy something to place in the bag, so that it wasn't just booze that I was buying. How sick and strange was I at the time. I'm still a little sick and strange today but I have the tool to deal with life. Pure insanity was about to start.

Once I opened the can of malt beverage, I took a long guzzle. I drank it as quickly as I could. I wanted to get wasted, I wanted to escape my troubles.

I didn't know at the time that I was about to cause myself more turmoil by not being honest with myself. This destruction was going to create a bender that would last weeks. I spent the rest of the night listening to music and having foolish conversations with anyone on social media that would talk to me.

I drank, I drank, I drank; then I cried myself to sleep that night. The next morning all I wanted to do was drink again. I noticed that I had an extra malt beverage in the fridge… so that is what I had for breakfast that morning. When it came time to check in with prerelease later that day, I lied to the caseworker.

Once I was able to "trick" my caseworker again. I became so sick with just isolation and depression that I played a cat and mouse game with them. I wouldn't skip a check-in then I would drink after, maybe they should have done house visits with me. Honestly at that time, I was not thinking clearly. I had just finished a nine month "drug binge" and was arrested on some serious charges. I didn't care to even be out free anymore. I was doing nothing productive; I was isolation and secretly drinking in my apartment for days. The days became weeks and it got so bad one day when I couldn't even afford the cheapest malt drink in the beer cooler at the store that I drank mouth wash for a week. Now that is some nasty shit, damaging to the body to.

I became extremely codependent in those nine months doing massive amounts of heroin and cocaine mostly before my arrest. I didn't realize at the time, but I was hanging on to Charlie like a drug as well. Thinking back to how I started this massive down fall has been difficult today.

During those months I had made no contact with my son and the daily pain of that is what kept me doing more and more drugs or a drink. I was running away from this mess I had created by leaving an unhealthy relationship suddenly. Although it was something that I wanted; I didn't realize at the time that it was a major life change. This major life change was a difficult transition for me, I didn't realize it at the time.

I tried to cover the pain with using any substance to not feel the real hurt in my heart, the pain of not being there for my son. My ex had placed a protection from abuse order on me and I couldn't have direct or indirect contact with my son. So, I gave up trying all together.

I felt as though I wanted to just give up on everything at that point because I was alone. Charlie was still in the jail, and I was left to take care of everything left in the apartment. I decided to place everything in storage and just turn myself in to the jail. I had no money for food, I had no money to pay the rent. My landlord placed a thirty-day notice to quit on my door. I ripped it off and just threw it on the floor. When I think back to those days, I can remember that I was lonely and spending all my time waiting for Charlie to call. When he did call it was late in the evening when I was inebriated, I was mean to him on the phone, and we argued.

Eventually one day after a night of drinking, I had to check in to the jail. This time I was still half buzzed from the night before. She did alcohol strip in my mouth and failed it. I was booked in the jail for a couple of days. Then the case worker decided to give me one more chance to try to get my life in order.

Honestly, I did want my life to change, I wanted to be free from what I was doing to myself, but I had no clue where to start. I would be set free from the jail once again just to start the self-pity party once again. I was in such a bad frame of mind that I was trying to "forget" what was really going on, in such a denial state of mind.

All I thought about was using any substance to numb out, to just forget about my troubles. Instead of trying to figure out a plan, I was trying to figure out how I could further destroy myself.

The saddest part of this part of my story was that I could have received help from my community. If I only had reached out and surrender myself. I was not ready; nobody could force me to be ready.

A few days after I was drinking again, this time straight vodka with no food, no chaser. Just plain vodka for days. I came to a point where I woke up with shakes every morning, the only way to rid these shakes was to drink. The days turned in to weeks. I decided that I had enough. I had a warrant out for my arrest and I had not checked in with the prerelease for weeks. I wrote a letter to Charlie, letting him know that I had left everything in the apartment all except for the photo albums, along with a few sentimental items. I stated in the letter that I wasn't doing so good and that I'm turning myself in to the jail.

The night that I turned myself in to the jail was the best thing that I could have done at the time. My body was so sore from daily drinking with no food. After I was locked away for months, the prison took blood work to see if I cause my organs any damage. I very surprised that all my blood work came back normal. Pure insanity is what I refer to these days now. Once I was booked into the jail, I asked to see the nurse, I informed the jail that I had been drinking for weeks. I was able to see the nurse at the Bangor jail, but I wasn't given any medication. The jail placed me in an area of the jail where they kept all the drunkards. I beat my body up so much that I felt as though I was hit by a bread truck,

I felt my body craving the poison once again, I needed medication. I thought back to when I was at the Knox jail and how they treated me, so kind compared to this joke of a jail. Once the guard walked by me, I waved to him to come see me.

I heard the loud metal door open, It felt like I was in a dungeon in a castle someplace foreign. Once the door opened, I said to the jail guard, "My charges are from Knox County not Penobscot." The guard just looked at me as though I wasn't important. Then I said to him, "Please, call them to get me." I knew that I would at least get medical attention at that jail. Once he locked the door back, I felt so sick to my stomach that I rushed to the toilet with dry heaves. I felt dizzy and almost collapsed. I knew I was close to a possible seizure. I curled up in the steel bed with the fuzzy blanket, then cried myself to sleep. This is when I started to pray, I prayed that if I survived this that I would change my life and change the path.

I looked up to this dirty cell wall and I asked my higher power to help me I whispered, "Please, Great Spirit, help me to see what I need in order to get well; I promise that I will dedicate my life to helping others." I felt this feeling in my soul that I had come to a point where I was ready to do something to change my whole life path.

Next thing I heard was "Paul, sit up. The nurse is here." They called you by your last name. Not sure if that's done purposely to make a person feel as though they are not human or just protocol. I sat up slowly, the nurse checked my vitals. She asked me a whole bunch of questions. I was as polite to her as much as I could possibly be, then I broke down in tears. I cried to her, "Please give me something for the discomfort, I feel like I'm going to die." With the tears rolling down the side of my face, she looked over at me then said in a soft voice, "Melody, I will help you. Please stop doing this to yourself." I wasn't exactly sure what she was telling me. She said to me, "There is a twelve-step program that has helped me. She was trying to tell me something. This was a fellow addict/ alcoholic, the message was clear, there is a solution to your madness.

Then she handed me the medication, I swallowed it as fast as I could. Back then I had experimented with needles, so I crave the shot of one desperately. Taking the medication calmed my nerves slowly. I laid back down then fell back asleep for a few more hours, my body was craving the sleep. Then I heard another knock at the door, and the guard said to me, "Paul, gather your belongings you're getting transferred." I was so happy to hear that, imagine being happy to be leaving a jail just to go to another. I gathered everything that they had given me. I was so excited to see the transport guard from Knox County. I said to him, "I'm so happy to see you. Thank you for picking me up so quickly." Lucky for me he was already in Bangor for a court hearing when he received a call to pick me up.

After changing back into my dirty street clothes, I was escorted to a car that looked more like an undercover sports car. I was placed in the back seat and handcuffed. Once the garage door opened, I could see the blue sky, it had just been raining outside. It was one of those weird rains when the sun comes popping back out after with clouds passing by. I felt this calming feeling as if I was surrendering my soul. I was just so happy that I wouldn't be killing myself slowly.

this is when I thought about what I had done to cause myself to be in this situation. This car ride reminded me of the times when Charlie and I would go down to visit his sister, only this time I was going to jail for furnishing substance to her. This shame and guilt came over me again I felt as though I couldn't take it. My heart was hurting thinking about my son, thinking about what a mess I created in a short time. I felt so shameful that I wanted to die, that was why I was drinking myself to try to "die." My addiction to substance had me on a rampage of self-destructive behavior for almost a year.

The feelings of uselessness and shame were haunting my inner core. I couldn't come to terms that I had something to do with causing an overdose death of someone that I cared so deeply for. A soulless act of selfish and sick behavior, that's what it was. I was sick and suffering, I had no clue how I could possibly change, I didn't know that there was a solution to my madness.

Imagine all the weeks I was drinking to cover this pain, when only I was just avoiding my problems just like before. The feeling in my heart was sadness for the beautiful soul that died due to my selfishness, just to get high.

After being booked into the jail, I was placed on a heavy dose of medication and placed in a maximum area of the jail. It honestly looked like an efficiency apartment, one bedroom with a toilet, the other room had a television set and a metal table with attached metal chairs. This is when I started to feel my mind coming back, I was detoxing my body. The nurse checked on me every couple hours. The medication I was given was a combo of drugs that made me feel so relaxed that I slept for days. I was placed in this max unit for observation and detox.

This is the place where I started to write down why, when then how... how could I slip up so badly to go on this year long bender of desperation. I couldn't except the fact that I had lost my time with my son, I couldn't accept the fact that I was in trouble with the law as well. Altogether I had caused so much pain that I figured the easiest way out would be drinking myself to death. How foolish was that game plan... this is called pure insanity at its finest?

I got to a point where I could be placed with other inmates, I was taken out of the max unit to join the other female inmates. I didn't really want to leave this private cell at first, because I had my own tv set with cable. I wasn't ready to talk to anyone especially other women. Back then I looked at other women as threats, only because of my insecurities. Lucky for me I was placed in a cell with a single bed for three months. In these three month is when I started my first book. I had hours upon hours to just write and heal my soul. Writing became my to go to, my comfort. When I was happy, I wrote, when I was stressed, I wrote. In every scenario in that jail is when I wrote.

After three months I was transferred to another jail called two bridges, I knew that I had been placed at the Knox jail by accident. I was a waldo county inmate not Knox County.

Looking back to these days has brought me back a bit not triggered too much, I'm hitting a meeting this afternoon. After a few days at this new to me jail, I was taken to court. This is when I found out how much time I would be serving. At this point, I was already incarcerated for three months. I was given fifteen months with no probation. When I was taken back to the jail, I remained there for another few days. During this time, I went to classes, meetings, bible study. Then in one of my meetings I noticed this one tall man, I looked closer…it was Charlie going with the male inmates to a group. This jail had several groups that all the inmates could attend.

I waved to Charlie, then he noticed it was me. I walked closer to the window to get a closer look at him. I waved again. I knew that I might not see him after I was transferred to the prison. On my last day at this jail, when I was to be transported to the women's prison, I noticed that Charlie was also in the lobby area. The guards were getting him ready for transportation to court. We were in the same room again. I said to Charlie, "Hey, so I'm going to Windham now, I got fifteen months." Charlie looked at me with this sad look, as though it was the last time, he would see me. I asked him, "How are you? Do you want me to wait for you when I get out?" He smiled, then replied, "Mel, I would love that." then I said, "Okay, I will try my best to get letters to you and talk with your lawyer." Then the guard yelled to us, "No talking." We didn't care we kept talking.

The guard looked over at me, then said, "Ready?" I said, "Yup." I glanced over to Charlie as I walked by him in the waiting area, then said, "I will wait for you, then get us a place." "Okay. I will write you too." Charlie's face lit up, then smiled, he uttered the words, "Melody, I love you. Please don't forget me." Then I said, "I won't forget, I love you too, Charlie."

I was able to see him right before leaving for prison, which I thought was very good timing. After I was placed in the van with the other inmates being taken to prison. I felt this sadness in my heart. I wanted to stay at this jail. Only because Charlie was there. I knew that I could forget him then move on.

Looking back on this time has made me understand why we needed to be apart. A person cannot heal completely unless they can focus all their energy on their recovery process. I believe today that this was the great spirt kicking in to guide us. Healing process.

Now where was I with the home buying process. After waiting for the all the paperwork to be processed of home buying. I received a phone call to let me know that all the paperwork for the underwriter was completed and ready to be approved. After all the running around getting everything in order. It was time to move, time to move forward. Time for change, change is especially difficult for the fellow addict. I have learned that alcoholics don't like change. I knew this change would be good thought. I didn't want to walk by people sleeping in the hallways, leaving old needles behind. I was ready to move into this house in a quite different neighborhood. I had been waiting so long to just be able to live in peace.

The day we moved we had all the boxes ready. We had rented a moving truck and a few people from the recovery community helped us move. It took us about three hours to move all our boxes. We decided to leave behind a love-seat and bed, in case there was any bed bugs. That apartment had these nasty bugs before, but we had kept up with spraying out apartment with bug spray regularly. I didn't want any bugs to hitch a ride to our new to us forever home. I bought two new beds for us, one for us, one for my son's room. A few hours after everything was unpacked from the truck, I realized that it wasn't a dream. That I had done this, I had done the work my credit counselor suggested. It took me over a year to make the payments to pay off the banks that I owed money. I had used checks to buy a few groceries but mostly just wanted cash back to buy drugs back in 2016.

I also had to work diligently to raise my credit score. This meant cleaning up my side of the street, cleaning up all wrong doings during my active addiction days.

The saddest part is when a person isn't ready, they are not ready to stop. They do just about anything to continue the war path of self-destruction, self-sabotage.

My credit score was in the low five hundred when I started working with this nonprofit agency in Orono, Maine. They had me check in once a month, with everything else that I was trying to do this was one of the appointments that I would not miss. Cleaning up my mess was so far the hardest thing that I had to do. Looking back at shameful behavior was pure torcher to me. There was a lot of shame, guilt, embarrassment that I caused.

Standing in my house with unpacked boxes, I thanked my higher power once more. I felt so proud that I had a house, a house that was mine. A private place to settle into and really start my healing process. My recovery journey had brought me this. If I hadn't surrendered myself, this accomplishment wouldn't be possible. If I was still drinking or drugging, I would be more focused on that. This is when I felt such calmness in my core again.

For the first time in a while, I slept like a baby in my new home. It was incredibly this newfound freedom from the apartment life. I wanted to yell from the top of my roof, "I WILL BE OKAY AGAIN!" As crazy as that would be I just settled myself in a healthy routine again. I was able to attend my meetings and do my facilitating at the Thursday Wellbriety meeting at our local recovery center, just minutes from my place. This was a special meeting for me, only because I was able to connect with native people in recovery on a spiritual way. This meeting is my favorite meeting.

I was introduced to the Wellbriety movement through an organization that helps native Americans in the state of Maine. I first went to my first Wellbriety meeting back in 2012, when I was in a women's rehab. This is when I met a few special friends. The facilitator of this meeting was a native American Author and local musician in our area, his name was Allan s. I had seen him before in and around native gatherings, but I didn't take the time to introduce myself and conversate. I can say that our first meeting together is when I knew I had comfort in this recovery circle of new friends. The other special friend that I met that day was Dominic L, he would always have a warm smile when I entered this meeting, which made me feel so welcome as a newcomer. At this meeting is when I first started to speak and share my experience strength and hope.

I continue to get to this meeting weekly, I wanted to feel connected with my peers. This was when I knew that Wellbriety would be a huge part of my story.

Another special friend that I would like to tell you about is Pete H. I first met him during one of the outside park meetings in Bangor. A group of recovery friends started meeting outside during COVID because all the local places "shut down" like everything in the world during that time in 2020. Pete was one of the new recovery friends that I had met during COVID at these outdoor meetings. Pete was very open and honest about his journey. I knew that he was one of the serious ones. Once I went to a few meetings and talked with him about my recovery journey. We would soon become close friends; he would regularly check in with me during the week. Pete was a healthy fit middle-aged man, he enjoyed working out, so I would take walks with him.

One day just before the meeting started, I was talking to Pete about something... then I remembered that it was his birthday. I said to Pete, "Hey, brother, happy birthday." His face lit up slowly almost turning red then he replied, "Thanks, Mel, I appreciate that especially coming from you." I then said, "You're welcome. What are you doing for your first sober fiftieth birthday?" He looked at me, then said, "Mel, I was thinking of going to have dinner downtown Bangor someplace. Would you like to join me?" It warmed my heart knowing that I had the pleasure of being invited. I said to him, "Can we invite a few of our friends from our group?" He said, "Absolutely, Mel."

After the meeting, I looked around for Pete, I didn't see him running off. I noticed that he left without giving me hug so I mentioned it to the group of our friends that it's his birthday and he's planning to go downtown to have dinner. There was me Charlie and a couple others from our group that went to this sports bar downtown to see if he was there. Sure, enough he was just sitting by the bar, drinking water and waiting for his appetizers to arrive. I walked over to him. "Pete, why did you just leave?" He said, "I don't know. I thought you guys didn't care." I gave him this serious smart face. "Really? Well, we do, and we are here so let's get a table, okay?" He looked at me and smiled. "Thank you for coming to see me." I didn't think that it wasn't a safe place to eat. I mean for an alcoholic to be sitting at the bar area of a sports restaurant was a bit sketchy. We all were seated in a nice area of this sports bar; everyone was drinking either water or soda. It was a very good recovery after meeting dinner. I had never done that before, only with Charlie and my son.

After dinner, we ordered Pete a cake then we sang him happy birthday then took some photos and shared on social media. We all filled up on good foods and extra chocolate cake on our plates. This is how we celebrate with food.

I had a lot of fun that night, our food bill was expensive but well worth the memories we made. After that I had a good friendship with Pete. Then a couple weeks after that we all went out to have dinner again. We became close recovery friends. He told me of stories of when he was growing up and he read my book as well. Pete told me that he was interested in writing a book, I told him I could help guide him along. I considered him to be one of the people that I could call and just talk about anything, we were friends.

I tried my best to stay in touch with him over the winter months, checking in on him like I do with some of my close friends. Someone in our circle had told me he had "gone back out," which usually means using substance once again. I called him one afternoon during one of the craft fairs I was at with my books in Ellsworth. Once the phone rang a few times he finally answered. I said, "Hi, Pete, I'm just checking on you today." He replied, "Hi, Mel, I'm just peachy, girl." That's when I knew by his voice that he was either drinking or on a substance. We talked for about twenty minutes that day, he wanted me to visit him, but I knew that I wouldn't be a good idea for me. I knew that I could relapse if I just let my guard down even just for a minute. It can happen that easily, I have relapsed a few times. Sometimes for me it involved two different types of temptations.

A few days later while in a hardware store looking for something for the house. We had just moved into the house, so we were still getting things organized and unpacked. I heard my phone ringing; I went to answer it. Someone in my recovery circle was calling me that never calls me, this is when I had a bad feeling. The person on the other line was calling to let me know that Pete had passed away of a suspected overdose. My heart fell to the floor, I felt anger and sadness at the same time. I wanted to yell again at the top of my roof, NO, NOT YOU PETE. I know how it gets when a person is in active addiction, it honestly is there choice to stop. Even if I went to see him when he asked me to… I asked myself, *Would that have helped? Probably not.* I had to come to terms with it. It took me a few days just to get my thinking back to my reality, my reality was that I couldn't numb out the pain with drugs. My medicine was recovery support and as many meetings as I could get to.

After a few days, Thursday rolled around so I decided to have our meeting dedicated to Pete. He was our friend, our brother, our recovery family. I announced it on my social media page, so I had a few new faces that I hadn't met before come to share about Pete. We placed a chair in the middle of our circle that day in honor of our brother Pete. We also had a moment of silence dedication for him. I could feel this energy in the room that day, it felt as though his spirit was there with us in the room.

Honestly, it's almost been a year now since he has passed away, I still think of him daily. I remember his energy and the passion he had for life. I loved how Pete would always say exactly what was on his mind at that very moment, not holding back, no sugar coating. He was a very intellectual Man with a lot of skill in his words. His love for adventure was contagious, his quick wit was always intact. Pete h was my friend, and I will always keep his memory close in my heart.

When I lose people in my life that I have let into my heart, it does make me want to go out and use every substance I can think of. Today I choose not to pick up because I know that I could not come back from my minor self-abuse state. This is exactly where I have messed up my recovery in the past. Something happens and I didn't know how to handle or deal with it, so I "numb out instead." I don't want to numb out anymore. I don't want to "run away." I want to work through my feelings like a normal person, but this is the part where I tell you… "Surprise, I'm not normal, I'm an addict and alcoholic." I'm far from the normal person. I have a disease that I must continue to medicate with meetings and recovery community, or I can die.

I used to drink for days and days without food or proper care of myself. I used to go days without sleep while I was high on a substance. I used to self-sabotage my life on a regular basis, because I hated how my life was going. Getting wasted and acting foolish wasn't good for me. I won't go back to that… especially not today.

When I decided to turn for the recovery road, I gave all my trust to the great spirit. I surrendered myself not only to the prison system but to give my life a chance to change inside and on the outside. I had to adopt some faith and trust in my higher power. I knew that I was killing my soul slowly for years, I didn't have the energy for this lifestyle anymore. It was time for me to make some major changes and to keep them in line with discipline. Step three.

This is when I started to pray daily in a room, mostly I would find a quiet room where I could not only stretch but to tell the great spirt how I was that day. Not saying it out loud but just in spirit. When I pray in the morning and have my spiritual time, especially early in the morning when everyone around me is still asleep is when I feel the most peace.

After accepting the fact that I had to continue to move forward in my life. I knew that my brother in recovery Pete was in a better place. As desperately as I just wanted to get angry and self-sabotage my life. I had a bit of anger toward this disease but what would that have solved? Nothing, it would have helped nobody. It was my disease telling me to quit the recovery life and go on this massive bender. I knew that I had some people in my life that would be hurt if I had gone that dark road again. I had just moved into my first house. I was getting my life in order; I was helping others in recovery. I knew that I had to really had to talk to someone besides my therapist. This was too deep; I couldn't bury it. I knew this is when I needed the help of someone that knew how to guide me through this rough patch.

I went to see my sponsor "Ana," I knew I could get this craziness going on in my head under control with some guidance. At first, I messaged but that didn't help so instead of beating around the bush about it. I just picked up that heavy phone and called her for help. The phone rang just twice, then I heard a soft voice 'hello my friend, how are you? … It took me a moment to answer. I had already told her that I thought he had relapsed a few weeks before, then I said, "Hey, so remember that special friend I told you about that was using?" She replied, "Yes," just in her tone I already knew she knew. I said to her in a down voice, "He's passed away and I'm feeling very angry, sad, lonely and mad again." it took her a moment to find the words maybe trying to help me, so I didn't freak out some more. She replied, I'm so very sorry my friend, I know your hurting, this is what happens sometimes when we are in recovery." we had a long conversation about what has happened since I got sober and why we might lose people during this journey. Relapse is and can be deadly, it's not a joke, it's a very serious part of a deadly disease that really needs to be treated with care and comfort.

After talking with my sponsor Ana about it she suggested that I focus on self-care. I buckled down for a couple of weeks. I didn't lose sight of the fact that I had a program and community that was always there for me, no matter what.

This is the reality of this sickness that I have. A disease that wants me dead daily. If I don't treat this disease with meetings I could fall flat on my face again, with a chance of not getting up.

I recentered myself I started to just get more leeway this way. I had a book that had been released during COVID that I really didn't take the time to do much with. I had wanted to do many book signings but because we were all under restrictions, I couldn't do anything. I started to write this book. I was thinking at first that I would just do a revise edition of the first book, but I had a close friend tell me just do a new book. I knew this could be a major challenge, I was afraid of failure. I didn't want to just have a book out there that was going to possibly just hit dollar stores everywhere. I started off fresh and here it is.

A month passed by I knew that I my heart was healing, I was loving having a new house. I couldn't believe how peaceful it felt. How I could just go to my mailbox and not have anyone there asking me if I wanted to buy anything, like they did at that apartment. Listen don't get me wrong; I was very grateful that I had a chance to get on my feet. That's what I had to do, I had to start some place.

I attended more than three meetings steady for at least a couple months. I went on Zoom if I didn't feel the need to be out. The Zoom meeting really has been a gift during COVID. This new lifestyle was making it easier for me to juggle and balance myself. I didn't want to fall so instead I placed some major tools in my backpack this time. Some of those tools are trust, acceptance, faith in my higher power.

Moving forward after a friend passing was very difficult for me. Although I was already seeing a counselor on a regular basis, I was having trouble with coping. So, I turned to what had helped me before when I needed comfort. My recovery people, my community, my sponsor, my twelve-step program. I was able to talk about it and understand why sometimes some don't make it in recovery because the disease gets too powerful. Trust me when I say this, my disease has challenged me. Even when I thought I was safe, it comes to shines its ugly head to the surface. I beat it down with a little bit of emotional help from my recovery family.

The day that I knew I could count on these recovery friends is when I knew I wouldn't have to face challenges alone ever again. When I felt the most support is when I walked into the hallways of a recovery group, then basically emotionally let all my built-up anger out, "emotional throw up."

I didn't feel like I wanted to use substance to cope with this loss. I wanted to get past this hurt I was feeling deep in my heart. If I wasn't clean or sober, I wouldn't care how I dealt with the loss.

In the early mornings I enjoy my morning mediations / prayers. This helps me figure out what I will be focused on that day. I've been able to re center myself this way for almost four years now. I read a elders mediation book that I like to go by. Sometimes this reading tells me that I need to sit in silence to hear my higher powers direction. This is also the time I like to thank the great spirit for allowing me to live another day on this beautiful earth.

Getting past the pain of loss has been the most challenging for me in these first few years of recovery. I have had to deal with hurt the same way a "normal" person would. By sitting in the hurt and accepting that I can't change anything or anyone.

The best way I've been able to move forward was to accept, of situations that I can't control. I could have answered that last phone call I received from Pete just days before he passed, but I was protecting my recovery. I must do this today, especially if I believe a situation or place could potentially cause me harm or even death. When they told me remove yourself from people, places, things I listened. It's the tools needed to survive out here on the streets of an addict. Just like when a soldier has weapons during a war. We must protect ourselves and our recovery.

During my incarceration was when I really took a deep look into my life. I stared into a mirror that I avoided for so long, then asked myself why? I wanted to figure out why I was continuing to self-sabotage my life, time and time again. It was because I dealt with it by "numbing out" getting high, getting drunk or causing drama. I built a pile so high that it crumbed down fast when I took a minute to look at my behavior over the years. This is when I decided to take a deeper look at my own trash. A pile so large that I would take up a whole parking lot. Inventory work was needed, and I did the work.

I would have loved to just do some of the things that my peers did after high school. I went years and years living in denial over this. I was ashamed that I had these re accruing thoughts of self-sabotage that I couldn't really control, so I gave in…drank or drugged. I used every excuse that I could think of, I did everyone's inventory except my own. I looked at other people's mistakes, then made it my own, pure insanity.

I'm not ashamed to say it today. I can write to you and tell you surprise, I'm not normal, I have a disease that haunts me daily. A disease that wants me to lose, a disease that sit in the corner doing sit ups and waits until I have a weak moment so it can make its move. It's almost insanity if not treated regularly, the haunting thoughts of going back out to use "just one last time" will hit like there's no tomorrow. There are unfortunately people that can't or won't medicate the disease as regularly as they should, this is when the disease jumps in for the kill.

The following weeks I was still coping with this loss. I did what I had to do, I moved forward. I would sit in silence in the morning and pray. Praying for this pain to be lifted and make peace with it. I heard some old timers say on a regular basis the longer you stay in the halls, the longer you will make it alive. That's what I wanted…a new life, a new outlook, a better way.

I was slowly getting things right in my head. The old way of thinking for me was, thoughts of hurting or harming others, because I couldn't cope with my own trash is what kept me in the gutter for so long. Years upon years of denying myself the peace that I did deserve. I wasn't going to destroy my life once again.

I had published my first book, which sometimes made me feel less than because it wasn't a bestseller. Some people spoke negatively about it, some people loved it. The amount of support I received just from back home made me so happy to tell my story. A story of deep pain but finding another way to live free from my own sick ways.

When I struggled to be real with my recovery peers, is when I was secretly trying to self-sabotage. I had all these positive moments happening around me. Buying a house, publishing my book, having my family. All the good things going on, but still having thoughts of trying to ruin my life. It's not easy living day to day with this disease, its draining to the soul. Once I felt that my sickness is trying to make up a plan to hurt me, is when I hit the local meetings. I've made some real amazing supports these past four years.

I came to the realization that I can't control anyone that I love or care for. If a person does truly want to stop using substance, they will stop. If a person isn't ready, its best just to let go and let God. I truly started to change when I finally realized that my higher power had been there just waiting for me to come to my senses. That was years of self-destruction, not only did I harm myself during these years (mostly in my twenties) I hurt others.

I coped with a loss by getting support, getting to more meetings and being more open and honest with myself and others. It wasn't easy for me to talk about my own mess.

When I first took the steps to sit down and write about what was bothering my core. I sat down with my feelings and wrote down the exact nature of my wrongs, I wanted to bail out. I didn't want to look back on the harm that I caused people, I thought I would have to long of a list. This is what I was told would help me to start forgiving myself. That poor young teen that left her home just to start years upon years of self-destruction, harming anyone along the way. When I was a drunkard, I didn't care about anyone's feelings, they did come back to haunt me but only this time I had to fix it. I had to stop avoiding my pain and figure out why I was a mess for so long.

It's like having a butter knife and peeling an onion. Peels upon peels of trash, just to end up crying out all the hurt and pain. Pain that I not only caused myself, but I hurt others and anyone along the way. Mostly because I was projecting my own bullshit.

Adjusting into my new home, then having a loss in my recovery circle was challenging for me. I felt all these happy thoughts about becoming a homeowner. Then at the same time having this hurt of losing someone was weird and painful. I was like excited about everything I worked so hard for but at the same time guilty because I didn't want to forget my friend. I was headed for a lot of pain but just didn't know.

I made phone calls, I went to meetings, I stayed in close contact with my sponsor.

One day during my morning walk, I received a phone call from my friend Cadillac Bob. Bob never called me; I would call him. I heard his voice. "Hey, kiddo, how are you?" I replied "Hey, Bob, I'm doing what I've been doing, I'm stable." Then

I asked, "How are you?" Bob's voice went low. "Well, I'm not good. The nursing home is sending me to the hospital." I answered in a panic, "Why?" Then he said, "They don't know how they can help me anymore, Mel." That's when I knew he was taking a turn for the worse. Bob had been placed in the nursing home a few months earlier because he was having a hard time at home. Poor Bob didn't have a wife or spouse to take care of him. He was struggling living by himself, living in Jonesboro in a senior housing complex. I drove down to help him once every few months, cleaning his apartment, helping him organize.

I first found out Bob was sick with cancer when I noticed all the medication/ vitamins on his kitchen table when I first got out of prison, a few years back. I asked him why he was taking all the vitamins his answer was brief: "I'm sick, I have cancer." When I went to visit him in the hospital, Bob had lost at least twenty more pounds since I last seen him. Then due to COVID restrictions he couldn't have visit at the nursing home.

When I walked into his private room at the hospital, he gave me a half smile. I felt so bad for him. He was hooked to all these machines, one of which was oxygen. I held Bobs hand he couldn't really talk in his regular voice. He was mostly whispering because he lost his voice due to the cancer spreading in his body. He had a large red lump on the side of his neck. I knew that it was the cancer. I sat with him for about an hour. I told him how sorry I was that I caused him annoyance, and he said to me, "That was a long time ago, dear." Poor Bob, it was clear that he was dying. His skin was a yellowish gray; his face was sunken in a bit.

He was very happy to see me. I held his hand and sat there with him for a couple of hours. My mother was good friends with Bob, they had known each other since they were both teenagers. I called my mother on video chat. They were both so excited to chat with each other. I could tell that Bob was very happy to see my mother on the other side of the screen. They were able to talk to each other and reminisce about the old days. I told Bob I loved him then gave him a big hug and kissed his cheek then said, "I love you; I will be back tomorrow." He smiled then replied, "I love you too, kiddo. I see you soon."

The next day when I returned to the hospital. The nurse told me that Bob was put on medication to make him comfortable. I looked over to Bob, he was just snoring sound asleep. I sat there for about thirty minutes. Thinking he would waken to visit with me. He just lay there looking peaceful, so I left. The next day I received a phone call from the hospital telling me that Bob had passed during the night. They told me that, I was still welcome to come see him for a few minutes to say goodbye.

That was hard for me, I knew that deep down Bob was in a better place. He had suffered with his health problems for a few years. Now, he wasn't suffering anymore with the pain caused by the disease of cancer. I walked in he was there on the bed. He looked at peace, I sat down next to him where I sat the day before. I talked to him as though he was still alive. I said, "Hi, Bob, I can't believe you're gone. You were my best friend for so long. Who will take this place now?" I shed a few tears while I held his hand; then I kissed his cold cheek once again. I whispered to him, "I will miss you, Bob; I love you, please watch over me now."

I left the hospital that afternoon feeling this emptiness in my heart. I always had Bob to talk to because I trusted him. I don't think I trusted any like I trusted Bob. The pain I was feeling didn't make me want to drink or drug. It made me want to get angry and like I wanted to go into the spin cycle. I messaged my sponsor to let her know that I had just suffered a great loss. I was honest about everything, I told her that I was hurting but that I didn't want to drink or drug. I ended up doing something that I knew would only be helpful to me, that was going to a meeting to talk. I knew that I could vent out my feelings safely with my recovery friends. It's so helpful that I can't really describe the feeling I have after talking and listening to my recovery people.

This was the major test in my recovery, I had just suffered a great loss. Not only was it a loss but it was a loss of a friend I had known for twenty years. I do believe that if I didn't have a program along with the support of a fellowship, I would have lost my battle that day.

Moving on from that pain, I knew I had to just keep doing what I was doing. I had just started a rough draft of this book, so I focused on that.

I knew that I had some vacation time that I could use so I planned a getaway to Boston to visit my aunt Shirley.

She was someone that I cared for and wanted to spend time with to recuperate. She had messaged me to congratulate me on my book. I told her that

I could take the bus down to visit with her. I wanted my son to get to know her and to see the city as well. Anthony hadn't really experienced a real city before except for Portland. I planned the trip a month before, I booked a couple night's stay at a couple different places one in south Boston and another close to Dorchester.

I could have drove down there… but really, I just wanted to relax and enjoy the trip. I didn't want the hassle and stress of parking and driving in the big city. I just wanted and desperately needed a therapy / fun trip. It didn't take long for us to get there on the bus. The bus only stopped twice, for short periods.

We arrived at south station at noontime. My son was so excited to see the city, I wanted this visit to be a memory maker.

I called my aunt Shirley to meet us in downtown Boston. When I called to tell her of a meeting location it was going to be right there at south station. She mentioned to me that it would take her at least an hour if not more to get downtown from her place. Anthony and I looked for the nearest coffee shop mostly because we needed our energy level to get back up there. We walked around the streets of Boston, looking around the high buildings and checking out the people for at an hour then we found a dunk. It was so fun; Anthony couldn't believe how large the buildings were compared to what we were used to back home in Bangor.

I was used to Boston already, but I hadn't experienced in so long that it was almost new to me as well. I was in my glory walking around with my son in the big city. Smelling all the different types of food, pizza, Chinese, fast food, etc.…

Once we got our afternoon coffee fix, we were ready to get our sightseeing trip on a good start. My auntie called me to meet up with her. Shirley knew the city well; I knew that she could help us get around. Anthony and I walked back over to the bus station. I saw my aunt Shirley standing by the waiting area. I called her on her phone to see her reaction. The phone rang 'hello, melody? Where are you? I heard my auntie speaking our native language. I replied to her in Micmac, hello, I'm right in front of you can you see me now? we all started laughing.

Once she seen us her face lit up like a Christmas tree. We went over and gave her a hug. I told her we had just been walking around the city. We all sat down to figure out a plan, she knew of all the wonderful places we could show Anthony. I wanted him to experience and know that other place besides Bangor's, existed and I wanted to teach him that staying close to family is what's important.

We walked around the downtown area for a couple hours. We decided to go check in to the hotel where me and Anthony would be staying for the night. This hotel was in Dorchester, it was right near a beautiful beach and very close to the subway (train station). I booked that hotel just for that very reason, so we could take the local transportation easily. We checked into our room for the night, then we left to go check out the mall area around Dorchester.

I already knew where I wanted to go eat, I'm not exactly sure I can use the name so I will just write that it was a famous Dorchester family with the last name starting with a W. I wanted a big fat juicy hamburger with French fries and soda (pop). Once we walked into this place, the server was polite with a nice big smile. He asked us where we wanted to sit. While looking at the menus, we all joked around saying to each other, "what if the famous owner came to bring our food" we all laughed and joked around. My aunt always had funny jokes to say in Micmac and knew how to have a good time. Shirley and I always got along well and had a good laugh together. Once we were ready to order, the waiter came over I could remember his big smile and energetic vibe.

I ordered exactly what I wanted, juicy cheeseburger with fries and beverage. Once the waiter took my order, I asked him if I could leave a book for the brothers? He looked at me, then asked, "Book?" I replied, "Yes, my book." I showed him my memoir, and he looked a bit surprised. He then said, "Absolutely, I will make sure he gets it." I talked to this waiter for a few minutes, mostly telling him a bit of where, why and how long we would be in the area. After having our lunch, Seth, our waiter, came back over to collect the check said to me, "Hey, Melody, if you're going to be in the area in the next hour, you can meet the Chef Paul." I knew the chef was one of the famous brothers. I could feel my adrenaline rise, and I said to him, "Really?" With a big smile he said, "Yes, he happens to be in the area. He had to come here anyway. I told him about your book." I was so excited; my son and I were just filled with excitement.

Little did we know that we would have the honor of meeting a celebrity that day. Seth asked for my phone number, he said to me, "Stay close, okay?"

I just smiled at him, then said "Yes, we will just be next door." After forty-five minutes I received the call, it was Seth, the waiter, "Hey, Paul is here and would like to personally thank you for the book." I was so excited that we all rushed back over to the restaurant. I noticed both standing by the door of the restaurant. I whispered to my son, "Be assertive and polite."

I walked over with a big smile then said, "Hi, Paul, so good to meet you, I love your restaurant." He then replied with, "Thank you so much for the positive feedback. I'll be sure to read your book." I then said to him, "Paul, this is my son Anthony." He looked at Anthony, then said, "Wow, you're very tall. Are you a basketball player?" We all laughed. Paul then asked, "What brings you two to Boston?" I said with a big smile, "We are visiting our aunt Shirley." He smiled at us, then said, "Oh nice. Well, I must get back to work. Thanks again for the book." I asked him if we could take a few photos together. He was so polite and nice to us.

I had no idea that we would be so lucky to have the pleasure of meeting a celebrity that day. After that we looked around a few other stores, then took the bus back to the hotel room. We had been walking almost the entire day. All I wanted to do at that point was to shower and crash out.

The next morning, we had plans to check out the new England aquarium. I never had the chance to go before when I was a kid. I had already purchased my tickets online a week earlier. We took the subway train to downtown Boston. I felt as though I was a teenager all over again. Getting on the buses and trains in Boston took me back to great memories. This time was different though, I wasn't that broke teenager living in the projects.

Looking back currently as I write this new story has been good for me. I do have to say that I never knew I could be so happy being clean and sober. Having the chance to travel around with my son, experiencing cool moments like this. I thank my higher power daily for giving me another chance to live right.

Our second day in Boston, we spent the morning just walking around the city. We walked around just looking at all the different buildings in downtown Boston. Anthony and I were just having fun watching all the different people around us. I had a wonderful time. That afternoon we went to the new England aquarium made some memories with my auntie.

It's been nice to reconnect with family since I got sober and clean. Before I wouldn't care if I visited with family or friends. The only thought I would have if I was still in active addiction would be, where can I get more substance, so I don't have to feel. That's the insanity of this disease, the disease not only wants you to die but it also wants you to isolate from family and friends, the path it sets is pure destruction.

I not only have been able to reconnect with most of my family from back home in Eskasoni, but also here in the United States as well, my extended family.

After all the fun we had watching all the fish swimming at the aquarium, my aunt Shirley took us to Copley place. I have never seen so many stores in one area before, it felt as though we were in a maze of stores. My son Anthony was surprised at how many luxury stores there was in Boston. Boston is huge and so fun; it truly is my favorite city.

After a day of exploring the big city. We all went to eat some dinner, then call it a day. During dinner we all sat around joking around in Micmac. I gave my aunt a huge hug than we went our separate ways. I told her that I would visit again soon.

It's been almost a year now since I visited with her. I have COVID and I've been home from work for a week. I'm catching up some writing and other projects. Where was I… coming back from Boston It was a nice feeling knowing that I went on an adventure with my teenage son. Being a mother has brought me so much happiness. I wasn't ever able to take my son to do much when I was under the influence, I usually had too much time invested in getting "wasted."

That's the saddest part for me, when I look back at all the times when I caused heartache and grief to others. Then I had to take the time to either visit with them and tell the person that I was under the influence of substance, when I was either being rude. Being in recovery today the hardest part is when someone doesn't understand the disease. They assume that is how one behaves on a regular basis. During my active addiction I would do things that normally I wouldn't think of doing. Some examples are borrowing money, making up stories and excuses as to why I wasn't able to work or do something social.

Getting back from that trip made me realize that I had a good life here in Maine, I had a beautiful house to come back to. I had a job; I had a recovery circle of friends that cared for me. I had a lot of positives all around me. I was grateful to be back home, back to my routine, my safe space.

Getting back to work really helped me to establish a healthy routine and mindset. I enjoyed working at this industrial laundry mat. It was very draining at times but really after being in prison for a year, not much really bothered me. I settled back into a working routine. I did everything that my sponsor suggested that I do, continued to stay away from people that could cause me harm. I had times when I just wanted to go on a massive bender and self-destruct like inspector gadget. That would only cause me to back track all my hard work I put into changing myself. I knew that I was heading on the right path the straight path, nothing was going to stop me, not even my character defects.

One of my character defects is accepting the fact that I am a very sick minded person with many defects. One of my character defects is that I have a hard time trusting anyone. This might be my worst defect. I could have someone tell me that I'm beautiful and hit on me, but I still would think other things. Like I would think to myself, *He's only saying I'm beautiful to get something like sex.* Then I would tell myself, *I'm not beautiful.*

That is how my sickness starts in daily, thoughts of self-harm, thoughts of destroying my life once again. Regularly I think of bailing on my relationship. Thoughts of party with random men, thoughts of getting drunk at the local dive, thoughts of injection myself with poison once again. Thoughts like these can be managed by attending as many meeting and support services. The one thing that has become my most important reinforcement is that I get my smudge and I pray in the morning. I find the best time to shift my sick thinking is the early morning hours, when everyone is still asleep.

I sit down I pray to the great spirit that my thoughts will be calm and not self-harm today. Self-harm for me is thinking negatively about myself and doing everyone's inventory. I do believe that without my morning prayers I wouldn't be able to think positively. When I was in prison, I heard this saying a lot: "Do your own time." Well, it stuck with me, I heard it in my head daily especially when I was at work. Just minding my business at work is when I remind myself to breathe and do my own time.

A few weeks passed by I was back doing work, meetings, daily program of recovery. Things were good and stable. I was settling into my new home, getting it cozy and comfy. I had a space to write and start this new book that I'm writing now. Being able to do the things that I restrained myself from doing for years was freedom from self-sabotage at its finest. Recovery can be painful thought, especially when there is death of friends.

After losing someone that I considered a close friend Pete H, then losing a best friend of many years Bob N. This was a new pain all together, instead of just wanting to cry for days. I wanted to get angry and yell from the top of my lungs. Why, why, why am I being tested now? I wasn't ready to give up my fight to staying clean and sober. I wasn't ready to let go of my life. I wanted to keep going, I was having the time of my life just doing regular things. I wasn't running anymore from myself.

I had to come to terms with this pain of losing a friend, one from the disease and one from cancer. I was down deep with hurt feelings. I forced myself to keep moving, to just remain in recovery and all will be okay. I had friends that were struggling with the loss as well. It took me a few weeks to genuinely smile again. I knew that I had two more angels to add in my circle, my angels of guidance.

That's what we must do when we are in recovery, we keep moving forward no matter what. A battle is a battle, even if the battle is within us. The friends that we make during our recovery is sacred like a fire inside of us. When they are hurting or using their fire is diminished. Only when they get back to recovery the fire ignites once again. It's a process of healing the inner core.

After coming back from Boston, I took a few days off to regroup my mind. It was nice to see my aunt and spend time together. I find that I was able to travel just if I kept my daily prayers and structure nearby. I wasn't ready to make any other major changes. I just wanted to focus on my stability and recovery, body, mind, soul.

I had a few weeks to settle back into meetings and work and life. I tried not taking on anything that could send me over the edge. Deep down inside I was struggling just to remain calm and strong. I had a pain in my heart that wasn't healing fast enough, I was in mourning. I wanted to drown out all the pain with booze or drugs. I was stopping myself to jump off the deep end, I knew this wasn't what would help me. Instead, I neglected my health a bit. I started to comfort myself with food, I wanted to use substance by instead I relapsed with food. I stopped exercising as much as I could. I made excuses about why I was going to binge on food. Food was my addiction as well as drugs and alcohol. Anything that would mend this inner pain inside but not break me as much on the outside. I didn't realize it at the time but today when I look back it's something that I was doing to numb out a bit, food became my comfort once more. If that's what I had to do, then that's what I had to do, getting past the pain of losing friends was hard.

Then on the other hand I had these wonderful group of friends that I had become close with that asked if I would be interested in hiking up to Mount Katahdin as a recovery group. At first, I wasn't sure about this, to camp out together as a group was something that gave me anxiety just thinking about it. I had camped out alone before and with family but not with my recovery friends. I knew that I could be challenged by this activity. My answer at the time was yes, I can try to. I knew that I could bail out of it if I needed to, so that was like my backup idea anyways.

Weeks went by I just stayed the course on my recovery I did what I knew what was safe. I talked with my sponsor regularly about my daily challenges, I knew that if I had one bad day during this mourning period that I could erupt like a mad volcano. I talked about all the times when I wasn't ready; then I crashed and burned. I didn't want to hurt my recovery or my life anymore. I took baby steps with everything, especially during this madness time of mourning.

I took some time to heal my heart, I took the steps that were necessary for my mental health and for my overall recovery process. I can't close my eyes and not cope with everyday problems by just ignoring everything. I saw that I was slowing going in that direction. I had to shack it up a bit by getting myself to meetings and interacting with my recovery community.

Isolation for an addict can not only become a form of a bad behavior to groom their disease but a way to escape not dealing with what's really going inside. I personally at the time was dealing with both side of this pull. I wanted to be home and away from people, but I knew that could cause me to self-harm.

The only way I could get past this to move forward was to purge it out. Purging it out would be, talking with a sober safe friend or my recovery groups. Really the best route was just to be open and honest about my feelings of pain and emotional turmoil. I knew that was something that I needed to resolve. I was told by people in the halls that I needed to finish the process in order to have good standings with myself. I needed to focus on what I had done to cause my life to have these thoughts of guilt, shame, remorse, self-hate. I had to write down all the wrongs I had done to others but also wrongs I had done to myself.

Self-harm is a regular occurrence to a person suffering from this disease, it's almost like our escape goat. Our way of not "dealing with life" or "bailing out" from reality. A person that suffers from addiction is much different that the reality of a normal person. I personally in my disease have ruined my life because I had so much self-hate. Maybe I hated myself because I wasn't strong enough to stand up for myself when I was told to abort my first child. This pain haunted me on a regular basis in my twenties, so I drank or used substance instead of working on myself. This time around I knew that I didn't want to drink or drug. I wanted to cope with this pain in a way that wouldn't harm or damage me or others. I had to purge out this pain.

Summer months came, I had a friend from prison call me regularly. Her name is Amy; she was one of my friends from "prison," a friend that I would talk to about anything while I was incarcerated. I didn't spend as much time with her when I was "out" of prison only because she was still actively using substance, therefore I didn't spend as much time with her as I really wanted to. Amy started to do meetings with me in those first few months when she was freed from prison walls. We spend a lot of time together while locked up. During this new freedom from the walls would be different thought. She didn't seem as interested in changing her ways to adopt this new way that I was into. My road was recovery, she was actively using again. This is what ultimately tore us apart.

Amy and I had become close friends when we were both serving our sentences in prison. She and I just connected on the same level. I understood her language and she understood mine, it was awesome. When I first met her, I was playing cards with some of the other inmates. We talked about "home," which to both of us was Bangor area. We also knew a lot of the people from our area. I used to walk and talk with her around the women's center outside track. In the women's center there was sections which were numbered or called walks, which was a hallway lined with double rooms. Double rooms as in shared with another female inmate. There was bathroom with a few shower stalls as well. Everyone on our walk had a "hall chore," which was usually either cleaning the hallway floor or the bathroom. So, since I had no money on my books and nobody was sending me money, I was hired by a few of the women if I could do their chore for commissary. Commissary is anything that can be bought from the prison's "store." They had an ordering system, which inmates could order bags of coffee, bags of candy, chips, soda, shoes etc. I always charged a couple bags of instant coffee and creamer and a bag of candy, usually jolly ranchers.

There was plenty of ladies that didn't want to clean those bathrooms, I was all set for the month. I even had a few bags left over usually because I didn't drink coffee all day. So, what I did was I would usually end up lending people bags of coffee or creamer to get by until their commissary order came in. Amy was one of the first people to ask if I had an extra either instant coffee or creamer to spare.

The prison had the women's center for women and the pre-release center just down over the hill. I could see the prerelease center from our walking track. After getting to know her for a few months, she was transferred to the pre-release. Down over the hill is what some of the ladies like to call it. So, when a person is sent down, they are told usually that day, due to security reasons.

Amy came to knock on my cell door 'hey Mel, are you awake? I was just laying down usually reading. I looked at her "yes, what's up? She then said to me, "Well, I'm getting sent to down the hill," She was filled with excitement. Everyone in the women's center only dreamed of getting transferred to pre-release. Mostly because they didn't have a fence around the building and it was cleaner and more modern, also they were more privileges like smoking, working in the community, etc.

I gave Amy a huge hug and congratulated her because it was like an upgrade. Then she said to me, "Melody, maybe I will see you down there?" I looked at her and smiled, then said, "Yes, maybe." So, I gave her one last hug and told her to wave at me once in a while from the pre-release center walking track. We both laughed together. I knew that my chances of getting down there was already slim, my paperwork had already been classified to "max" for some reason.

After a couple my caseworker at the prison called me in to her office. She then said 'would you like to go to prerelease? At first, I wasn't sure. I only had a few more months until my release, so I wasn't as excited. I told her that I would think about it and give her an answer by the end of the day. The only reason I was as excited is because I had a structured routine at the women's center. I had my daily time typing my first book in their computer room, that was almost completed at the time. Also, I had made some good friends at the women's center over the months.

After talking it over with a few of my friends I went back to my caseworker "Jennifer" that everyone called "Jen" to talk it over with her some more. One of the major factors I didn't want to leave was this routine I built over the months. I liked the fact that I knew everyone at the women's center, I wasn't sure if I had the energy to try to get to know more people in just a few short months. Change is good and that's what I did need in my life, to step outside of my comfort zone is to grow, is what I had to tell myself.

When the day came that I was to be transferred down. I was told to "pack my belongings," which I did as fast as I could so I wouldn't change my mind. I had made some good friends at the women's center, friends from all over the state, women that I was in the pods with that I grew to love and trust.

One of the ladies that I got close to and recently went to her wedding was Elizabeth O, she was always there for me when I needed someone that I could trust to tell anything. She was always there if I needed anything too. One time she was helped me get photos of my son and Charlie, so I would have these photos to look at and hang on my wall space that I was given. Elizabeth's ex-husband had copied the photos from my social media account then developed. It was honestly one of my best days in prison when I received those photos of my family.

Some of the women I met in prison have a special place in my heart. Women that I still try to stay in contact with like sole sisters. Amy was one of those ladies, she was one of my close friends.

Once I arrived down to the pre-release center, I was very overwhelmed. Especially from the new faces, new set of prisoners that I knew nothing about. I did see some familiar faces, women that were at the women's center. Some of them I knew and talked with, some I just knew by face. It's hard to like try to get to know so many people and remember names. It's a different world in prison, it's a whole different way. One of the inmates that I was in there with at the time was working on a documentary about her life and struggles as a person living with substance use disorder. Her name starts with a J and ends with an H. The documentary was done well. I watched it for the first time yesterday.

Well, anyway, after a few days of settling into a routine I settled into a routine. I was a getting settled into a routine of writing, working out, meetings. One day while walking around the outdoor track I heard a familiar voice: "Melody, wait up." I recognized the bubbly voice. I looked around and it was Amy I said to her, "It's about time." We both laughed. We walked around the walking track outside until it was time to go back inside. We laughed and talked for hours about old times. Sharing our war stories and talking about recovery and how we both had a desire to change our lives. Amy was friend that I felt comfortable telling my deepest darkest wrongs. Amy knew a lot about recovery and how to get past situations that could be harmful. I would tell her about what wrongs that I had done over the years, the wrongs that I was shameful and guilty of. I felt as though she understood that I had a huge desire to change my life.

During our hours of conversations, we would share stories about life and our struggles. Overcoming self-hate is very difficult and it was absolutely very challenging for me to love myself once again. I focused mostly on my recovery process the most. Amy was always there to listen to me vent about all the minor stressors; I listen to her stories as well.

Basically my 5th step.

We talked about future, like when we got back home which was Bangor to the both of us. That we would start to attend meetings and do things together in the community. She talked about our struggles, and we told each other the truth. She was my friend, and I loved her soul.

After I was released from prison, I did everything that I had thought about doing. I found a landlord that would accept the fact that I was a felon and gave me a chance. Honestly, I had a friend in recovery introduce me to Andy (landlord). The nicest landlord I've ever had.

I found a job that I didn't mind (coffee shop). I started to go to the local meetings and participated in the meetings. This is when I got serious in my recovery process, I listen to the old-timers a lot.

Amy got out a couple of months after me. She called me a few times when she was still in prison. I wrote to her and gave her my information. I wanted the change that we talked about during our walks and time together. Because really in prison the only thing you can dream about is change. I had this desire to jump as far as I could without my disease of addiction coming in the way of it.

I invited Amy over to my house for coffee and show her my new apartment. She was so proud of me for getting back on my feet so fast, I told her that I had help getting into the apartment because I had been discriminated against because I was a felon. It wasn't easy to get to where I was at the time. I wanted to help her, and I told her that I would go to meetings with her regularly. That afternoon her boyfriend came to pick us up and we all went to the local recovery center in brewer.

Afterwards they dropped me off back at my place. Amy and I stayed in contact regularly after that. We talked on the phone regular, and I did go and visit her when she moved out to dexter.

Unfortunately, I had to let her know that I couldn't visit as often as I would have liked to. The deadly disease of addiction got the best of her. I had to listen to my sponsor was telling me. I had to take care of me and protect my recovery. She understood when I told her that I had to be distant because I have my days too. I wanted to remain clean and sober, and I couldn't have people in my life that were using.

When I received a call from her in the hospital, I was worried. I told her that I would support her recovery and always be there for her to sit next to. I loved this woman; she was my friend. She had been drinking too much, her organs were struggling. She told me how scared she was to have this certain surgery performed on her. She was at the danger zone of the alcoholism; it was causing her poor health.

Although it was hard for me to tell her that I think she needed to stop substance. I told her that I loved her and wanted to have her back in my life as a friend in recovery. She got out of the hospital but continued to use substance. Then in Aug 2021 she lost her battle with the disease.

I was heartbroken, we had already lost so many people during COVID that it was just numbing. My heart was hurting. The insanity of the disease wants us to die and hurt so we could fall. As painful as this was to endure, I knew that I had to keep moving forward. There was nothing I could have done, and I had been reaching out for months.

This week was a strange on for me. I had a recovery camping trip all planned. A trip that one of my recovery friends was planning. We were planning a trip up to Mount Katahdin as a group. This plan was to camp for a couple nights in a campground and practice our daily recovery program as well, meetings in between and everything. The camping trip I told you about earlier was this one here.

So, it was just bad timing maybe, but I had already promised my friends that I would join them. Even though deep inside I didn't want to go. I was still in shock about Amy and really, I wasn't feeling like having fun, I was sad over her death. Everyone in our group knew that she had passed. That first night of camping I told the group that I almost changed my mind and stay home instead. But I decided to people please instead, a huge mistake on my part.

I talked about the pain I was going through, honestly, I couldn't help but be sad. To lose friends while in recovery was difficult to deal with. I had a struggle just to smile and that's not me. I love making new connections. The first day of camping was fun, went swimming with a few friends. Then setting up our camping area for the night.

The next morning, I wasn't sure if I would be going anyplace but home. I didn't wake up until seven and for me that was late. I didn't sleep well at all the night before. I drove to get myself a coffee to think about the day and to clear my head. After getting back to the campground, I noticed that some of my friends were ready to attempt to hike up the mountain. I was in decent shape so I knew that my body could handle it. There would be the five of us going up. We drove to Baxter state park.

I knew that I could have some challenges along the way, I was going to at least try. It wasn't too bad at first. There is a beautiful place back home in Eskasoni that everyone calls "the cross." It takes about thirty minutes to get to the top of this steep hill, then at the top there's a huge white cross. That's what this climb feels like but instead four to six hours incline up the mountain. There was me and carmen, the two only females. Then joe, Andy, rick. We all said a prayer before starting our journey.

I had my best trail shoes on, just in case. I dressed in comfort as well.it was mid-august so all of us were dressed lightly. We all knew the weather was calling for some rain showers, that didn't stop us. Once we started our climb, I would occasionally look at the view behind me. It was so beautiful up there on the mountain. A couple hours passed by; we all were doing good. Everyone had packed extra waters and snacks. After about the third hour hiking, it started to sprinkle a little. Then at about the fourth hour it was a full down pour.

We decided that we wouldn't chance it, especially hearing the thunder roaring. Walking down that hill, I took a few moments to enjoy the beautiful views. Then once we got to the bottom, we were all soaked from head to toe. I think we all were ready to nap by the time we got back with our other friends that decided to do the smaller trails. I felt a bit defeated, and I wanted to just go home.

When I got back to the campground, that's what I planned to do. I just wanted my own bed. Charlie was the waiting with the others. We had a disagreement and we got into argument instead. I think that I created this drama in my own head just to 'escape 'my disease was talking to me. Instead of talking about it I held back and exploded. I left the campground to "cool off" but instead I had rick call me to tell me that Charlie was flirting with a woman in the campsite area. I was so upset; I drove 25 in a 5-mile zone. The campground owner came over and asked me to leave. Honestly, I was already packed and ready to go.

So, I used a non-sweet voice and told him, "I'm already packed, and I would love to leave." Then he rudely replied, "Then go." Charlie and I drove off but before we crossed the town line in Millinocket, the police pulled us over. Charlie and I were in a heated argument and I was very upset. The police asked if I was hurt or in danger. I said, "No, I'm not in danger, but I really just would like to get home. The police took both of our ID cards and ran our names then let us go. I was so upset on the drive home. I felt so embarrassed about the whole situation.

Once we got back to home to Bangor, I helped unload the camping gear, then changed out of my clothes. I didn't tell Charlie where I was going because I was still so angry. I wasn't sure where I was going but I knew one thing that was on my mind…drinking or drugging.

I was sitting in my car at a coffee shop, calling a few "old friends." It's like I was waiting for the right opportunity to sabotage my life. It's almost as though I played out the drama just so that I could go use substance. Lucky for me none of my "old friends" picked up the phone that day. Otherwise, I might not be writing this book right now. Then I called my friend Dom L, I knew he would pick up his phone. Once I heard his voice, I started to cry. Sitting there in the parking lot I was telling him what had happened and that I felt as though I might be leaving to party. Dom knew what to tell me at that exact moment so I wouldn't go back out. He gave me an earfil of good advice, then said call your sponsor.

So, after I got off the phone with him, I called Ana. She too helped me with her kind words but also reminded me that it wasn't worth going back out, that I needed to slow down and breathe. I felt better after talking to both. They helped me to understand that my disease wanted me dead and that was why I created this scenario in my head. I was hurting inside over the pain of losing three friends just months apart. Little did I know there would be another hit to my heart just months after this one.

The reality that the alcoholic /addict is weak without the proper medication. Medication that includes meetings, community, friendships.

So instead of going to drink or drug that day. I drove to the drive through window and I order myself a milk and doughnuts. Another addiction of mine that can creep in from time to time, food addiction. This is when I decided that I needed to go back home like a "big girl" and talk about why I was so upset. Talking about things that bother us is very important. If we allowed "things" to stay inside of us. We actually causing ourselves more trouble in the long wrong.

This is when I decided to have my higher power remove all my defects of character. Step six.

I prayed on the drive home, I prayed that I would have the strength to carry on, let go and let God. I wanted to leave the life I was slowly building once again. I was trying to Relapse, or self-sabotage is the reality of it. This deadly disease wants us to give up and sabotage ourselves. Its cunning powerful and baffling to say the lease. I had these sick thoughts of just 'taking off', like when I use to when I was actively using. Even some of the old behaviors come back from time to time, especially when I don't attended meetings and open to others in the program.

After talking to Charlie about our 'camping trip', we came together to talk. We talked about how we both still needed to focus on the program. Living with another addict can be overwhelming and extremely difficult at times. I told Charlie that I should have stayed home instead of trying to "people please" so that I wouldn't let my recovery friends down. This is when I knew that if I ever needed to just stay home to breathe, then that is what I will do.

I prayed to my higher power that day, I asked him to remove all my short comings.

After a few days went by I decided that working and reaching out to others for help would benefit me the most. I wanted to focus on this Recovery Path that I was walking and continue to help others in my recovery process. I knew I had to work on some more personally issues after this 'camping fiasco. I wanted to get all my demons out so I could just live like a normal person, the reality is that I'm not normal I'm addict addicted to everything and anything that blocks my reality.

I thought about when I was in prison, when I was locked away for my irresponsible and insane behavior. I wrote so many letters to people that I had harmed or hurt. I wrote a few to my family back in Eskasoni. I wrote letters and sent them out in the mail to a few people. I also wrote letters to people who were no longer here on earth, including Charlie sister Georgiana. I wrote to her letting her know that I was so sorry for the pain that I caused to her family. I wrote that I was sorry that she was no longer here on earth. I also made a promise to her that I would change my path and help others in recovery.

I knew that I had to mourn the loss of the friends that I lost. I took a few days off from work just to selfcare. Just to understand that death is a part of life and that I believe they will be my friends in the world after this. I also took some time to just be lazy and do nothing for a few days. That is what's important in recovery to just selfcare. To just breathe and take a step back and eat some ice cream and watch favorite movies for a day or two.

I knew that I needed to regroup myself especially after the pain in my heart for my friend that I lost. I focused on service work and writing for a bit. I knew that I had to be extremely careful, or I could fall hard. When I realized that I couldn't stop myself from crying anymore and let go of the hurt, this is when I started to feel again. After the process phase, I realized that I had more work to do on myself.

When I started to figure out what was bother me inside, I knew I had to instantly get rid of it. It can turn into disease really quickly if you allow it to just sit, sit and do pushups. The terrible disease of addiction can turn a good day into a sour day as quickly as the weather changes in new England.

I focused most of my energy to homework, working, helping others. That's why my friends always encouraged me to do. Sometimes we lose friends but gain new ones along the way. Changes are extremely uncomfortable in recovery; I know this especially to be true.

When I noticed that I was missing a void in my heart, I decided that I would get a dog. I wanted a smaller breed dog. I reached out to some local animal shelters but I they didn't have small dogs. I looked in the newspapers and other sites in my area, no luck. I decided that I would do my research on social media. I found a breeder that was located just an hour north of me in island falls Maine. The puppies were a mix of Maltese and Yorkie—a Morkie. I messaged the breeder to ask if they had any puppies left and when they would be ready to take home. I was in luck when the breeder said to me, "I have two left, a male and a female." That's when I replied, "I can place a deposit on the male, please."

I sent a money order out that very same day. I knew that having a puppy would bring comfort to our home. My son was having some difficulties at the time being a typical teen. I knew this would be a good thing for all of us. The love of a pet is therapy. The puppy "Buster" wouldn't be ready to take home until October the breeder informed me. Buster had to stay with his mother to nurse some more. The breeder (Greg) told me that the puppies were born August 15, the same day as Charlie's birthday. That's when I knew that this little puppy was a gift from above.

I started getting things ready for Buster's homecoming, which was still eight weeks away. I bought his bed and dishes for his food. I bought a few different types of toys that I thought he might like. Just knowing that I had a puppy on the way, I felt good inside. It was like I was getting ready for a baby but instead a puppy. I always liked the name Buster for a dog, I just find the name to be cute.

I called to check on Buster every couple of weeks. Greg was very professional and sent us photos with updates as well.

After a few weeks past, the camping trip helped me realize that I still needed to work on myself. Even thought I was approaching three years in my recovery, I still had issues that needed to be addressed. I decided that I would reach out to some of the people that I hurt in the past. Like my old boss Connie, Connie was nice enough to lend me money for rent back in 2016. I decided that I would start to send her monthly instalments of that "rent loan." Connie and I had a good relationship when I worked for her back in 2014. We had long conversations with her about everything that I was going through, her feedback always helped me stay grounded and focused.

When I was incarcerated in 2018, Connie wrote me a few letters and sent me a couple cards. I will tell you that when a person is incarcerated and they received mail, it's like a gift. I only had a few people write me when I was locked up in prison. Honestly when I would get any mail, I was so happy to even get anything. I cried once when I illegally received a letter from Charlie once or twice.

I was able to just stop and write a nice letter to Connie, I thanked her for giving me job when I was just getting back into the work force. I was able to write her a nice letter stating that I was a changed person in a way that I had never been before. I stay in contact with her even today.

Moving forward was on my mind and I knew that I had a few more letter that I had to write and either personally deliver to whom I had caused pain and hurt. I did write another letter to one of my ex-boyfriends and I decided to personally deliver this letter to Fairfield Maine. This letter is to him was directly from my mouth. I wanted to tell him that I was sorry for how I use to behave while highly intoxicated back in 2001 when we lived together. Back then my disease was in high gear, I had no responsibilities and it showed. I would just rent rooms because I was too irresponsible to get a regular apartment., because I was feeding my disease regularly.

I wanted to be free but I didn't know how to live, I had no program back then. I had no clue that I could live another way. I thought that living was working, then partying afterwards. Partying until I blacked out isn't really what I think is fun these days.

When I went to visit Todd in Fairfield, he was happy to see me. I messaged him on social media at first. Todd always treated me well. Our conversation started with how we were doing and what we had done over the years. He was doing well, and I was excited for him. We talked for a few hours, and I ended having lunch with him. Todd is a very special friend of mine and I care for him and consider him a friend. Before I left, I gave him a copy of my first book, and I wished him well. He told me that I could stop in anytime I wanted to just escape my reality. I haven't gone back since.

Once I knew that it might take me a little while to try my best to make peace with old friends that I might have caused harm. That was work that I was willing to work on. I knew that it was a process, and I was willing to just do what I needed to do for myself.

Processing and expecting my past for the wrongs I had done to myself, and others was very emotionally uplifting. I felt as though I was cleaning my side of the street. Only this time I was trying to make things right. Eventually I will call the campground and apologize for speeding. Working on my behavior is still a working progress. I can say that I still have so much work to do on my character defects. I understand that there are people out there that don't like me for the pain that they don't know how to process. I use to be that resentful angry person that couldn't target exactly what was troubling me.

Anyways back to my story. When I decided that I would celebrate my recovery time with another fellow native American. Someone that I considered one of my best friends. That was Dom L, he was someone that I had known for about ten years. I first met Dom back in 2012 at the native center that everyone calls "The Wab." Dom had this passion for sharing his story with me. This is how I was able to open to him about my trouble in life. This is how we connected at first.

I would see him around town when I was out walking in downtown Bangor. I knew that when he was out walking around town is when I knew that he was getting some mother nature medicine, like myself. We always talked every chance meeting, on the street or at the library. Dom used to tell me, "Mel, I just love the library, there is so much knowledge there." We always shared laughs together. He sometimes would joke around with me about something that only natives would understand, this is the part that I loved the most. When a native tells another native a joke only, they could comprehend is when it's even more funny. I know this sounds silly, but I bet you have met someone you could just laugh with. Well, this was me and Dom, he would give me a certain look at either a public place or at a meeting, then we both would just smile at each other.

Dom had this excitement about life that was just electric. He knew exactly what to say and at the perfect timing. Sometimes when we both were feeling a bit down, he would tell me, "That's just life, kiddo, it's not perfect but at least we are clean and sober." During one of my drunks, I called Dom when he was working for a local cab company in Bangor. I needed a ride back across tow, I knew if he was working that I could just pay him back if I was short on funds. He would make me priority and come get me then make sure I was in my apartment with the doors locked. The next day I would call him, this is when I knew I would get a slight lecture. In my drunkard stage I didn't know I got home, he always would leave me a message stating, "Melody, don't drink so much. You called me for a ride home and I almost had to carry you…brat." I knew I needed to call him and talk it over with him, I would always thank him with some food. Either we went out for lunch, or I would make him something. I knew I was safe with him, he treated me like respectful. When I really got to know him was when I was in rehab back in 2012. We went to a recovery meeting together. Sharing our stories of struggle was always a good learning experience for the both of us, opening up is very challenging for an addict-alcoholic. Sometimes it can be crippling to just say a sentence. Then over the years both of us relapsed a couple of times, when either one of us was trying to stay sober. Then only this one time we both were in "relapse mode," both of us had secretly starting drinking without talking about it. I met him on the street when he was on his way to the store to get a malt beverage in the early morning hours, that's what I was doing too. We ended up drinking together at a "friends" place later that day.

I slipped back into active drinking and using heroin for the first time ever back in 2016, he noticed that I stopped going to meeting and knew something wasn't right with me. I called him to borrow some money, he said, "I don't mind lending it to you, but I know what you're up to." Once I got to his place I fessed up and told him that I had recently tried the "H" and I hadn't stopped not even for a day. This is when he would give me one of his lectures. Dom always tried to help me out any way he could, I would help him out too. He was someone that reached out to me over the years, showed me that he cared.

He always would drop everything he was doing to help me. When I was actively using substance, he was the person that I called for a ride to the emergency room when Charlie was there for an overdose. That was when I was in the zombie zone. Then when I got out of prison Dom was there to help guide me to get my butt to meetings. He encouraged me to start the Wellbriety meeting at the barn in 2019. I would usually walk to the meeting alone, then meet him and two other native brothers, we always would sit together. That made me feel so comfortable in those meetings, knowing that I was not alone in the fight was very powerful force for me to stay clean and sober.

Then for the first time in a long-time Dom was coming up in a year of sober time. I knew that it was a big deal for him to get that one year. I had already planned my celebration with a special drummer and sweet treats for the meeting. I knew that I wanted to ask Dom to celebrate with me

My third year clean and sober I was supposed to celebrate my recovery time in august but instead I decided that I would mention it to Dom that we could celebrate together. I wanted to celebrate with me he was one of my best friends in recovery. When the day came that I would ask him if we could celebrate together, was a good moment.

At first I was excited to ask if he would be interested in celebrating with me. Dom always stayed with me after the meetings; then I would usually give him a ride back home. During one of these rides, I told him about the puppy that I was waiting for and that Buster will be his name. Dom laughed then said, "Buster is a cute name." Then we shared a good laugh. He seemed a bit anxious about his first-year celebration.

So, I just came out and asked him, "Dom would you like to celebrate to-gether?" He gasped out, "Really, but I thought your celebration is a month before mine?" I then replied with a smile, "Yes, but I'd like to celebrate with you." I could tell he was so happy. I could tell that he was honored that I would delay my celebration with him.

We both mentioned having it at the park that day, on Thursdays since COVID started. In our area there was outdoor meetings held. When every-thing was shut down that's when local recovery people started outdoor meet-ings. I was having two groups on Thursdays back-to-back. The first meeting was at the recovery center, then the other meeting at the park. People just brought their own lawn chairs, it's a beautiful park that is in the middle of town.

Dom and I decided that the park would be the place to celebrate, fresh outdoors with recovering people, it only gets better. Usually, Dom was my steady helper at the meetings, he always gathered all the literature and would carry the box to my car. Dom was always there to support me along my jour-ney. Finally on the day of our celebration, it was rainy out, so we decided to change the location to the recovery center.

we had a good crowd of recovery friends and family to gather for this spe-cial occasion. A native American female drummer that drove three hours to sing for the group, sang her heart out and everyone enjoyed it. I could tell from the big smile on Dom's faced that he enjoyed the celebration. After the ceremony we had some cake and shared laughs together. A couple weeks later during one of the recovery meetings, I gave Dom a ride home. When I pulled into his driveway I asked him, "Dom, everything ok? he looked at me a smiled, "yes dear, everything is fine." Then I said to him. "Okay, I love you, brother, stay on the recovery path." Then he said, "I love you too, kiddo." Then I drove home, little did I know that would be our last conversation together.

When I first got serious in my recovery back in 2018. Dom had been in the halls for months, he even offered to take me to a meeting. It's very hard when a person first gets sober, the shame, guilt, remorse that was racing in my head when I first walked in to that first meeting. Then seeing a smiling familiar face just broke my anxiety. Just getting accepted into the circle of these meetings is a wonderful feeling.

I never really opened and embraced recovery like I did this last time. Dom was along the way; he was one of my biggest supports.

I had requested some time off from work, a week to be exact. I was planning to pick up the puppy and get him a little housebroke and build a bond with him. Also, it was my birthday week, so I wanted to just focus on selfcare and writing this book.

When I noticed that Dom was not at the meeting that Thursday I wondered if he was just visiting family back in Indian Township, sometimes he would take off to visit family for a few days. So, I figured that's where he might be visiting home. I also reached out to call him after the meeting but there was no answer. I tried to reach him on social media as well but then no reply for days.

The Friday when I started my vacation is when I noticed I had two missed calls. I didn't check my messages for a couple hours, because I took a long nap after work. I wondered why I received these calls. I was in the grocery store picking up a few things when my phone rang. It was my friend Sue. She's a caseworker at the center. This is when I knew something was wrong.

When I picked up the phone, I was literally in the checkout area with a few items of groceries in my shopping cart. I then answered, "Hello?" Then I heard Sue's voice. "Hi, Mel, I just wanted to let you know that Dom had passed away today." I was in shock at first. I felt like walking out of the store and just leaving my groceries, but I couldn't. I replied, "What? Why? How? What happened?" All the questions popped into my head. She told me what had happened, and I felt this heartache in my heart. I finished my shopping; then I drove home. When I got home, I told Charlie and then I messaged my sponsor, Ana.

I felt so sad for this loss, it's like all my friends were leaving me. I wanted to call Dom, but I couldn't because he was gone forever. He would now be with the creator, he was with the others Bob, Pet, Amy all of whom meant so much to me. I cried for Dom that day, I prayed to him too. I said in my prayer, "Dom, why did you leave me? Now who will I call when I want to take off? Will you please get me when it's my time as well, brother? I love you."

The next morning was the day we would pick up Buster, our new baby Morkie. We had waited so long to get a dog; it took months just to find him. Charlie asked me if I was okay on the long car ride up North 95 to island falls. I was still in shock about Dom, so I stayed quiet during the ride that day. I enjoyed the lovely scenery, there is a turn off so Mount Katahdin can be seen well. Then we arrived up to this small town of island falls. Our destination was to our new puppy Buster. He would be my therapy.

When we arrived at the breeder's home, the house sat on a piece of private property. It was so nice to drive in then have like two different breed dogs coming out of the house. Two pug dogs came along with a Morkie that was full grown. Then the cutest puppy I had ever seen came outside to the porch to greet us. That was Buster. He was a light golden color with a bit of grayish tint. He was maybe two pounds. He was so tiny; I feel in love instantly. He walked over to me, and I picked him up, I said to him, "Hi, baby, I might be your new mommy," then I kissed his head. He was so light and cute, image like a stuffed animal but alive. The couple that owned all these dogs invited us inside to sit and talk. I asked if I could use the bathroom, long car ride. When I went down the hallway, I noticed two young children in the other room, they had another Morkie in the room with them. That Morkie was "Ruby" that was a female, but I wanted a male, which was Buster, both were so adorable. They would reunited later.

Then, after talking with the owners for a few minutes, they told us what to expect from him, his daily routine, and what kind of diet he was on. I paid for the puppy then I received his vaccine paperwork. I was so thankful to have the little one beside me. During the car ride I had him sitting with me, he crawled all over me and then he rested behind my neck on my shoulders. He was so comforting that my heart ache for Dom lifted a bit. This new puppy felt as though it was a gift from my higher power to help me not be sad anymore about my friends passing to the other side. I knew that I had a new friend, and I was so excited about it.

The puppy cried a bit during the car ride, but it was mostly excited energy. Then getting buster inside the house, he pranced around smelling everything. Buster was adorable, I loved hoe he was so tiny. That first night home, he didn't want to sleep in his dog crate that was next to me bed. I let him cry for almost an hour until I couldn't take it no longer. Then I said, "Okay, buster, just this time because you left your family." I placed him on my bed, he bounced around us like it was play time. Then I had to say in a calm voice, "Buster lay down, sleep." Buster scratched the blankets as though he was digging the ground outside. Then after a few minutes he fell asleep.

After that first night, I felt a connection to this little dog. He was very smart and already house trained. We got Buster his own small fence in the front yard. I walked him to the park near our house. He could hardly make it, that's when I usually picked him up and carried him back home. Buster must have been trained to fetch back at his parents' house because he already knew how. It was so cute. I made a video, then shared it on a social media site.

Not only was Buster helping me cope with my mourning process, but he made me laugh too. He had this personality of a diva already. I looked into his little face and kissed his head, every time that I had a thought about Dom. That first week of having Buster home was definitely a healing process. I even prayed to Dom and said, "This puppy is helping my pain, brother." That is the absolute truth. If you are going through something I would suggest a pet. The therapy these little buggers have it can be so healing.

I truly understand why people say "man's best friend;" animals are so therapeutic.

As I write this part of my journey. I'm currently watching my friend Heidi's sober house in Millinocket called Breaking the Cycle. It's a beautiful sober-living house for women.

It was healing mode for me after I got my puppy. He was helping my heart heal from the destruction of myself. Today I must take a deeper look at myself and my own actions because I'm my own worst enemy once I feed the demon inside me. I choose to feed that caged demon with love and patience.

After a few months passed, I decided that I would continue to heal my core with writing and self-care. I had no clue where I was going with this book.

I knew that all these wonderful supports in my life asked me when is the next book going to be out? I had no clue what to say. The pain I turned into art.

I prayed daily to my higher power that I could move forward. I was anxious to find another job. I felt as though I craved change. I wanted to continue the road of recovery by either directly helping others or even just guiding them into the recovery process. I knew that I had a few friends that were going to school to become substance abuse counselors. Those long days at my last job helped me realize that I wanted to have a job where I could be in the community helping other addicts and alcoholics.

I started filling out job applications weekly. I had a few interviews with a few places, but my criminal record always got in the way of getting a job. Once they found out that I was a felon, then I was immediately rejected because of it. That was extremely frustrating for me. I found myself by mid-December almost giving up on my job search. I just stopped filling out job applications. I almost went back to my old way of thinking, but I didn't, I couldn't.

Then after a meeting with a few community members, feeling mentally fresh, my friend Erika approached me. She had been working for Wabanaki Public Health for a couple years already. She was the recovery support /outreach coordinator. Erika was the one to help me to coordinate the Wellbriety Zoom meetings during COVID. This is how I first met her. Back in 2020 when COVID first stared, the state was shut down so everyone was having Zoom meetings. That's the only way we could connect as a community, honestly, I didn't like the idea of Zoom meetings at first, but I had no choice. If I wanted to remain clean and sober that is what I had to do, Zoom meeting or risk my recovery.

She mentioned to me, "Do you have a resume?" I looked at her with a dazed and confused look. Then I relied, "Yes, why?" She then said to me, "Well, I would like to have you on my team." I wasn't sure at first, because I was scared to leave the stability of what my current job had for me, which was healthcare, dental, and benefits. I said to Erika, "Okay, I will reprint my resume and send to them."

I wasn't sure at first, I was afraid to change jobs. I wasn't sure I was ready to make that leap. As an addict-alcoholic I have learned that change is scary for us. I was scared. I sent an old resume at first, thinking that they would just reject me. This was my way of trying to avoid doing something different.

The alcoholic inside me was saying, *"make the change so I can act up."* I didn't want to jeopardize my recovery in any way. I enjoyed the stability of a regular full-time job; the daily routine was predictable. That is what kept me there for a few years, structure.

Then the following week after the meeting at Wab, Erika asked me if I could retype a new resume and that she could help me. That's when a light bulb went off in my head. "Do this for the community, give back and help others." Then I realized if I make this leap and fail, I can always recover. I finally made up my mind after talking it over with my circle. I knew that I could "try my best."

I wanted to finish this book first before I took on any major changes. I was almost finished. I wanted to have a book that I could dedicate to the friends that has passed but also writing was my therapy. Losing Bob was hard for me. I broke down at his funeral. Then losing one of my recovery brothers and sisters Pete H., Amy W., then my Native brother Dom L.—it was a huge challenge for me to not drink or drug. During COVID we lost many brothers and sisters to the deadly disease of substance use. I wanted to share and help the fellow addict-alcoholic that you don't have to pick up no matter what.

Since I was an addict-alcoholic myself, I know today that I want to shout to the world that we are not bad people. Our disease wants us dead. Without the 12-step program I would not be writing this book. Without the help of friends in the community I would be isolated in an attic apartment once again. I don't want to die; I want to live life and help my people heal. Heal and guide others to freedom from self.

Today Buster is doing well. He is almost eight months old. His sister puppy Ruby lives in the area and they connect every few months. It's very cute watching them play. My son, Anthony, is doing very well in school in Bangor and working part-time at a pizza shop near our house. Buster is doing well and has all the comforts a dog could have. He's very spoiled and I take him on walks with me daily. Charlie just had major heart surgery yesterday and is recovering well. Charlie has been there for me with the first book and then now this second book. Charlie has grown in his recovery process and just wishes that he would have found recovery years ago.

I personally am doing better than I have ever done in my life. I have my struggles as a person living with substance use disorder. I keep a very close eye on my balance and recovery process, I stay connect with my recovery community. I stay in regular contact with my sponsor, she is a wonderful woman of worth and one of my best friends. Sponsor, thank you, I love you. I continue to facilitate a 12-step meeting at the Bangor Area Recovery Center on Thursdays. Come check it out, everyone is welcome.

My family back home in Eskasoni is very supportive in the life I live today. My hometown showed me so much support in my writing. I will be visiting them this summer/fall. I'm very grateful that I have found a newfound freedom and tools to figure out how to cope with challenges. I accepted the job at Wabanaki Public health, and I love what I am doing. I'm stable. Today I am happy to be clean and sober.

Wela'lioq- Thank you

The next few pages contain poems that a few of my friends have written.

Passamaquoddy and very Proud
of his American Indian roots

Big Heart, big smile, could be a little loud,
Was our friend Dom Lacoote

Dom's time on earth was much too brief,
Yet while he was here, he touched many others,
His death in October 2021 was met with grief,
We'd lost one of our very dear brothers

Lost as so many to this disease, never entirely breaking free,
recovery seemed only to tease,
Showed only a glimpse of what it could be.

His big heart for others was always full,
Bringing peace part of his walk on earth,
yet from somewhere else came another pull,
That seemed to constantly pull,
that seems to constantly question his worth.
One-year celebrations, when hope took flight,
followed by times of dark night soul,
We pray that Dom is now bathed in light,
and the great spirit has made him whole.

–By Joe Bennett

No Longer Alone

Thought we journey with others on this road,
we can still choose to make the trip alone,
No one can convince us to share our load,
The desire has to be our own.

At first, we feel the need to explain
To apologize for this drastic change,
Unimportant then was our pain,
And the need our lives to rearrange.

But then the light begins to dawn,
And at first tt's true it may flicker,
but if I'm running this marathon,
don't have to engage, no need to bicker.

I can walk with you, my head held high,
Before no one do I have to crawl,
I no longer have to notify,
or explain my sobriety to all

it's not my place to judge another's walk,
for I see each day how much I'm flawed,
yet we need not see it as a roadblock,
but trust it all to the grace of God.

–Written by Joe B.

Not by Faith

My friend asked me to write, so I will do it my way. I'm just telling anyone that reads this to pray. Pray to God that you still have a chance. Because life is rough, and it is hard to dance. But focus enough and you can figure out in time. Don't let failure be inside your mind, it's not an option, if you want to succeed. But if you are focused and don't let distractions interfere, you'll get what you need.

Everything I'm writing probably sounds like you've heard it before. Maybe cause that advice has been around for years and you need to hear it more. Wake up please before it is too late

Somedays you need to feel good, because of a bad day. But does that mean you need to throw your life right away? So many people I have seen die because of a high

I notice their families and kids wonder why? Why they can no longer come home for dinner or tuck them into bed. It's pretty difficult to explain why they are dead.

If you are alive and reading this, you are not alone. I am an alcoholic and struggle with this life of my own. I just wish that you can take some advice from me before it is too late

You are a wonderful person, so many people love you, death by addiction is not your fate.

–By Dustin Daggett

Melody Rose Paul

I feel like I want to die, but I can't say why
I'm ready to meet the other side
I know I'll leave some people behind, but I know they'll be fine
I say this out of fear, due to the ones I see dear
I can only say I wish we had more to this day
I see death is near, and I'm not in fear
I don't know why I'm waiting for the other side
I see death coming from behind, and I'm hoping it catches me
I slow my steps, so I don't have to be here, death I do not fear, please come
for me here and now
I need to see the other side
I know there's no choice to see if I want to reside,
But sometimes we all have to die, so please come for me so I can fly
I want to be with my family in the skies, I'm sorry to deprive my family on earth
I don't know how to handle this hurt; I know it's sad to flirt with the idea of death
I believe I'm ready to let my soul rest, I shall let this world go with this last breath
I'm struggling to hear what's left, Lord "my son" I've always been here by
your side, it's not your time to die, "my son," I can hear it in your heart, that
thought is a lie, in time you will be by my side
"my lord" why is my life such a struggle, my heart feels as if its troubled
Life is like a puzzle, it takes time to come together, soon your happiness will
be on another level,
Believe in me and you shall see

–Written by James Sock

Cousin

Forever missing you, it's always going to last

Remembering the times, they went too fast

Your eyes be glistening when you laughed,

I'll be missing the past time we had

My heart full of pain, it's never going to the same

You always had our back and you never turned that on us

Now everyone is missing you, the family be reminiscence you,

wishing you still here

I know your guiding us from above,

it's amazing how you showed everyone love

It's a scary thought that you're gone,

but in our hearts your legacy will live on

It's going to be hard but the homies, we staying strong

My time isn't over I'm going to represent you sober

You're the reservation's big brother and I can't see no other

Praying for your mother, hoping to ease her pain

God bless the family that's left,

I'm going to hold the memory of you 'til my last breath

When I was lost and confused,

I could always count on you for the right advice

Know I'm crying looking at the heavens

 wondering why you can't be by our side

I know the creator has plans, I'm glad you're in his hands

Forever missing you 'til I see you again, cousin

–Written by James Sock

Spiritual Gardening

Spiritual gardening is when we are true to ourselves
In our garden, we plant the seed, it is put in the dirt, covered in darkness
When we start working on ourselves like we are a garden
We are able to find the light and give it the nutrients it needs with love and
forgiveness
We start to see the growth of planting good seeds, taking out all the dead weeds
With willingness and love and nourishment and patience
We can have hope to see the light that we need
So, we can start healing to
Keep living and watching our garden grow
When we learn to let go

–Written by Sebrena May Tomah

Heal having the willingness and courage to speak

We feel at this moment, we're at a low time and feeling weak

Everyone struggles as we have different stories that need to be told, don't allow your heart to turn cold

Learning to let go of the pain, change needs to come from within. Be true and vulnerable, it's okay to tell your story, it will help you.

Someone relates in some way, it will help change your own or their life that day, we need to not allow the hurt and pain to stay inside, we need to stop hurting ourselves and allowing it to hide.

When we admit our past mistakes, these are lessons we are supposed to take

We need to ask for help, we are not alone, find someone you trust, pick up the phone.

We are here together as a team.

One step at a time, commit by staying clean and sober

you will have a better mindset

Your life is waiting, and we are worth it to live a life and start over

–Written by Sebrena May Tomah

Wantaqo'tiey Alasutmaqn: Serenity Prayer

Niskam iknmui wantaqo'ti
God grant me the serenity
Kisiksua'tun tan'n koqoey
To accept the things
mu kisi sa'se'wa'tu,
I cannot change
Mlkikno'ti kwlaman
Courage so that
Kisa'se'wa'tis ta'n koqe'l
I can change the things
Nuta'q sa'se'wa'tasin,
That need to be changed
aqq nsituo'qn kwlaman
and the wisdom
Nentis ta'n teli istue'kl
To know the difference

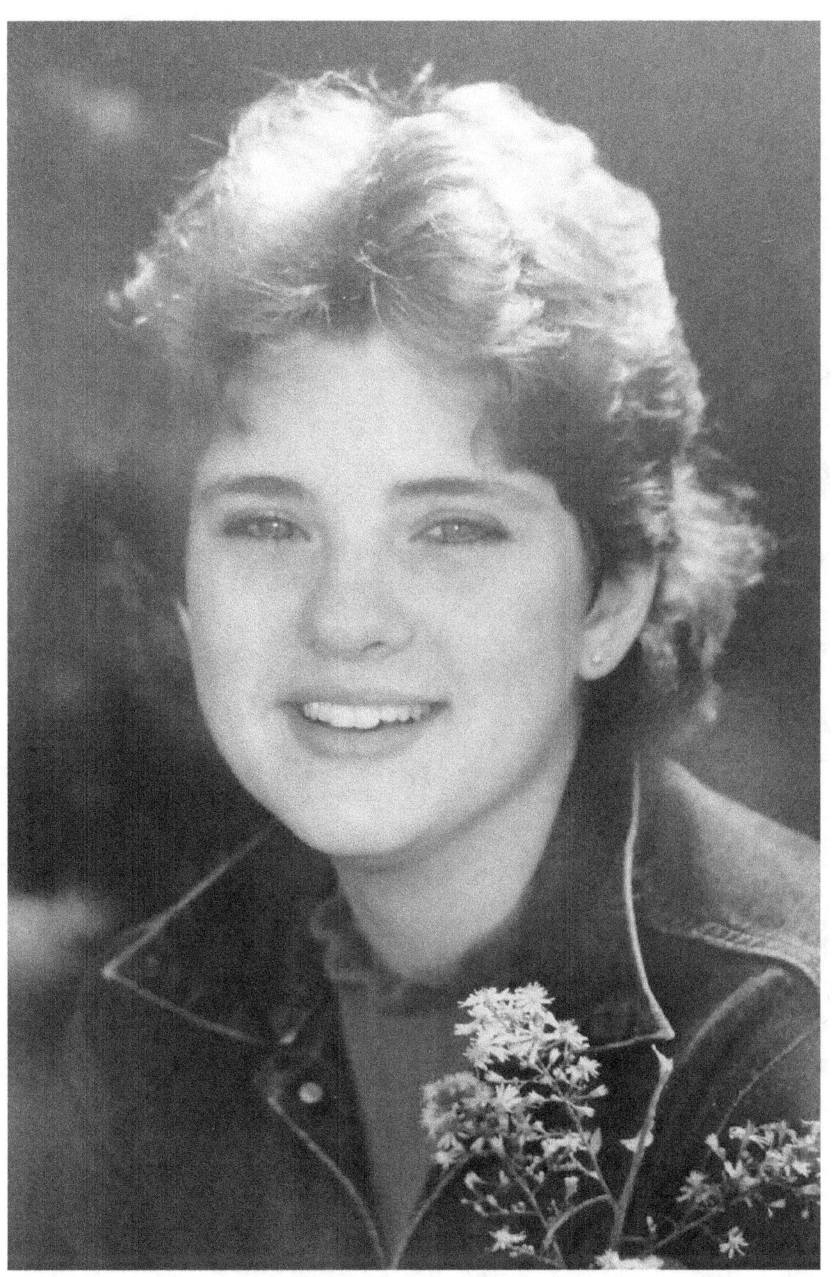

Georgianna M. Michaud
September 13, 1967 - April 6, 2017

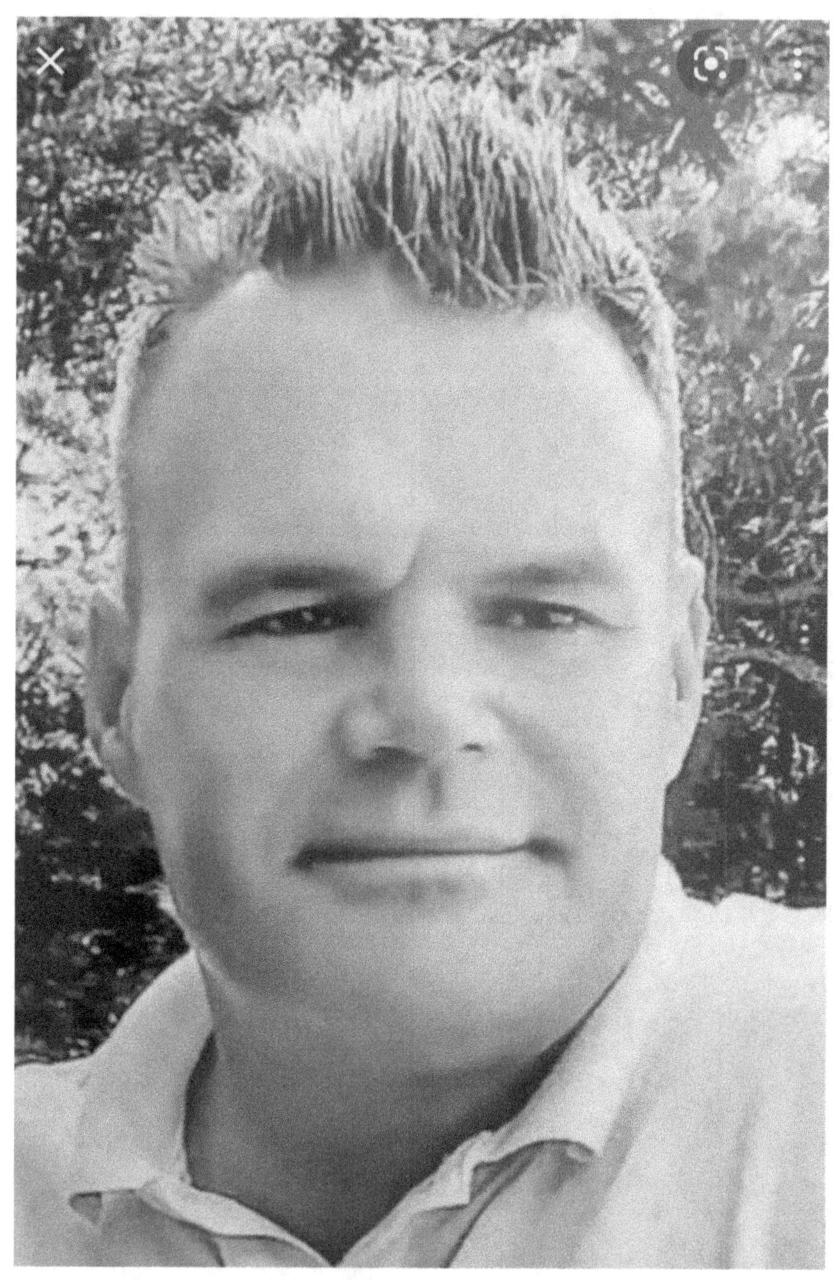

Peter B. Honey
October 30, 1970 - March 14, 2021

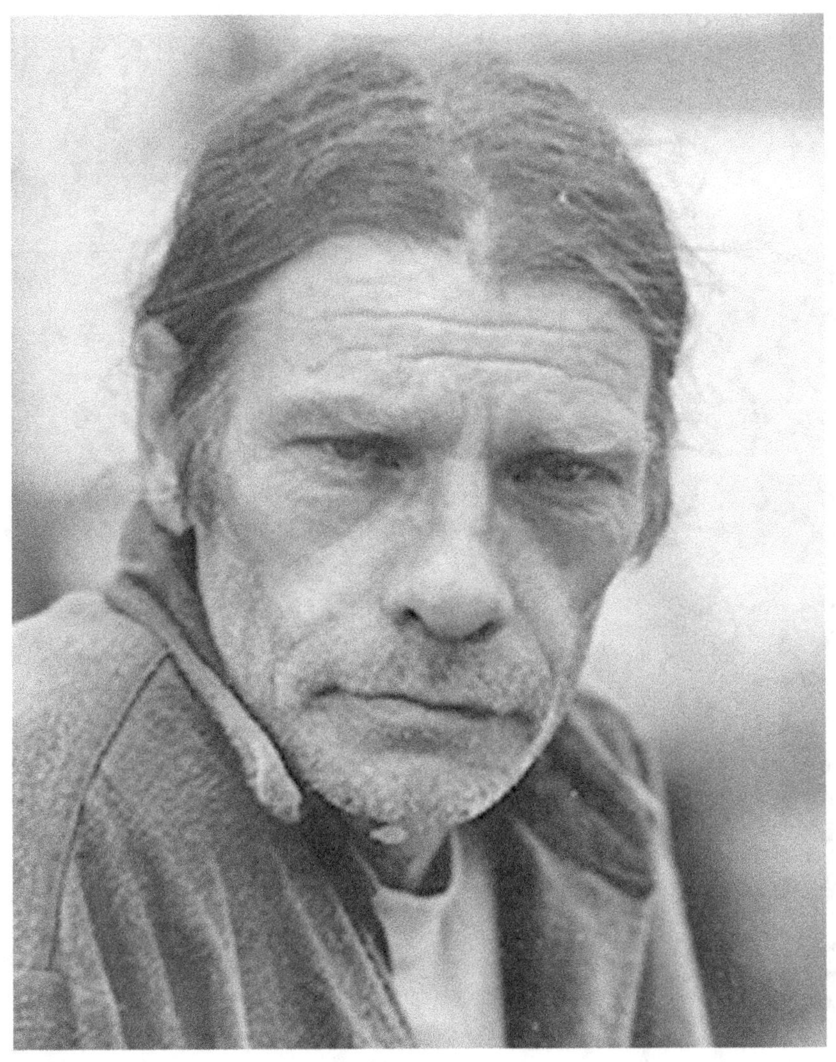

Robert Nichols (Bob)
June 1, 1948 - April 6, 2021

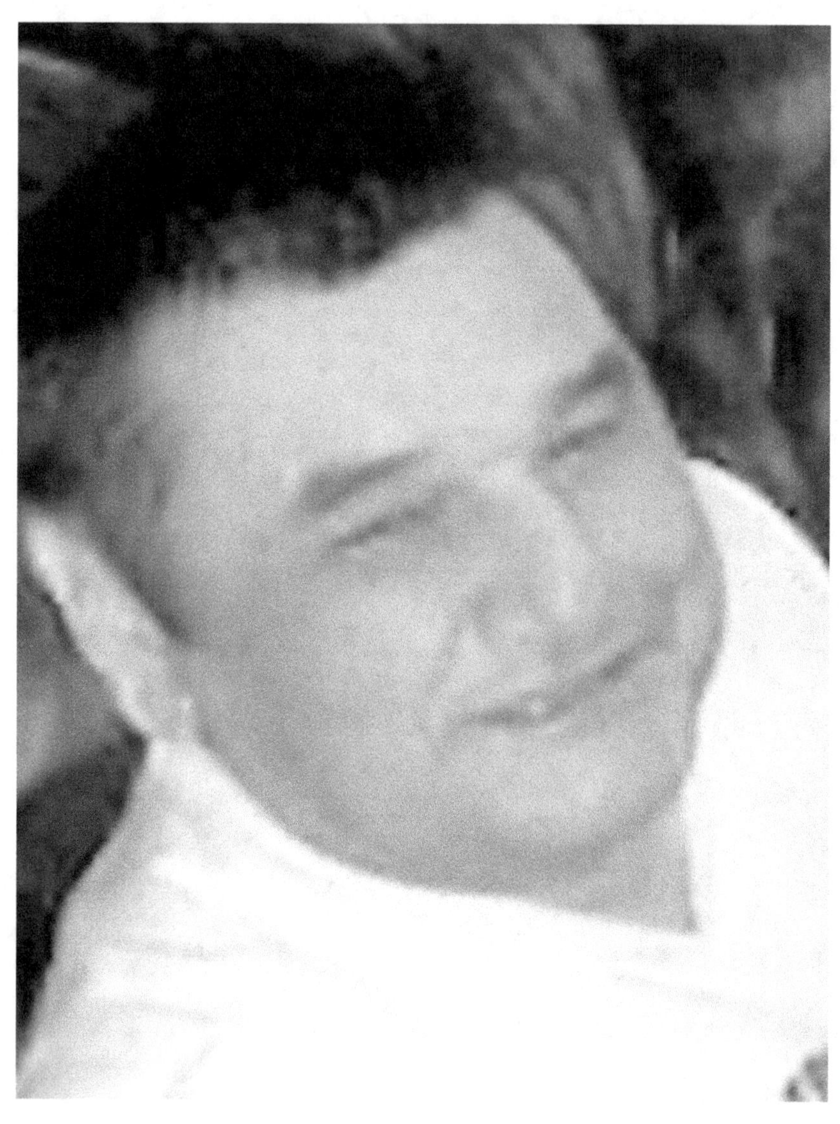

Dominic LaCoote
June 11, 1966 - October 8, 2021

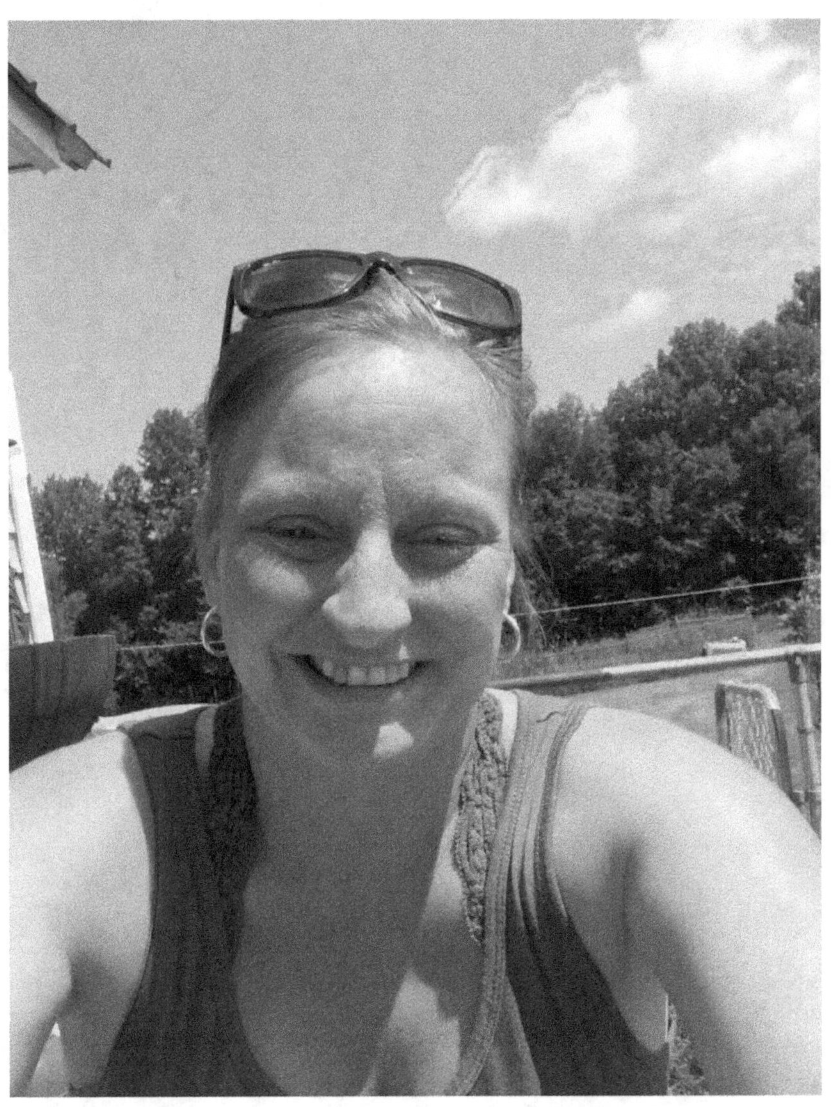

Amy White
April 21, 1976 - August 13, 2021